Welcome

Anxiety doesn't discriminate. No matter your age, gender, race, upbringing, or circumstances, anyone can suffer from it. Whether it's panic attacks or a debilitating disorder that stops you from living your life, this book is here to help.

Discover what anxiety is, how it can affect you, and the different ways of dealing with it. Then use the activity and journaling pages inside to explore where your anxiety comes from and how to work your way through it.

From practical advice to coping mechanisms and techniques, this book will guide you through your journey to overcoming anxiety.

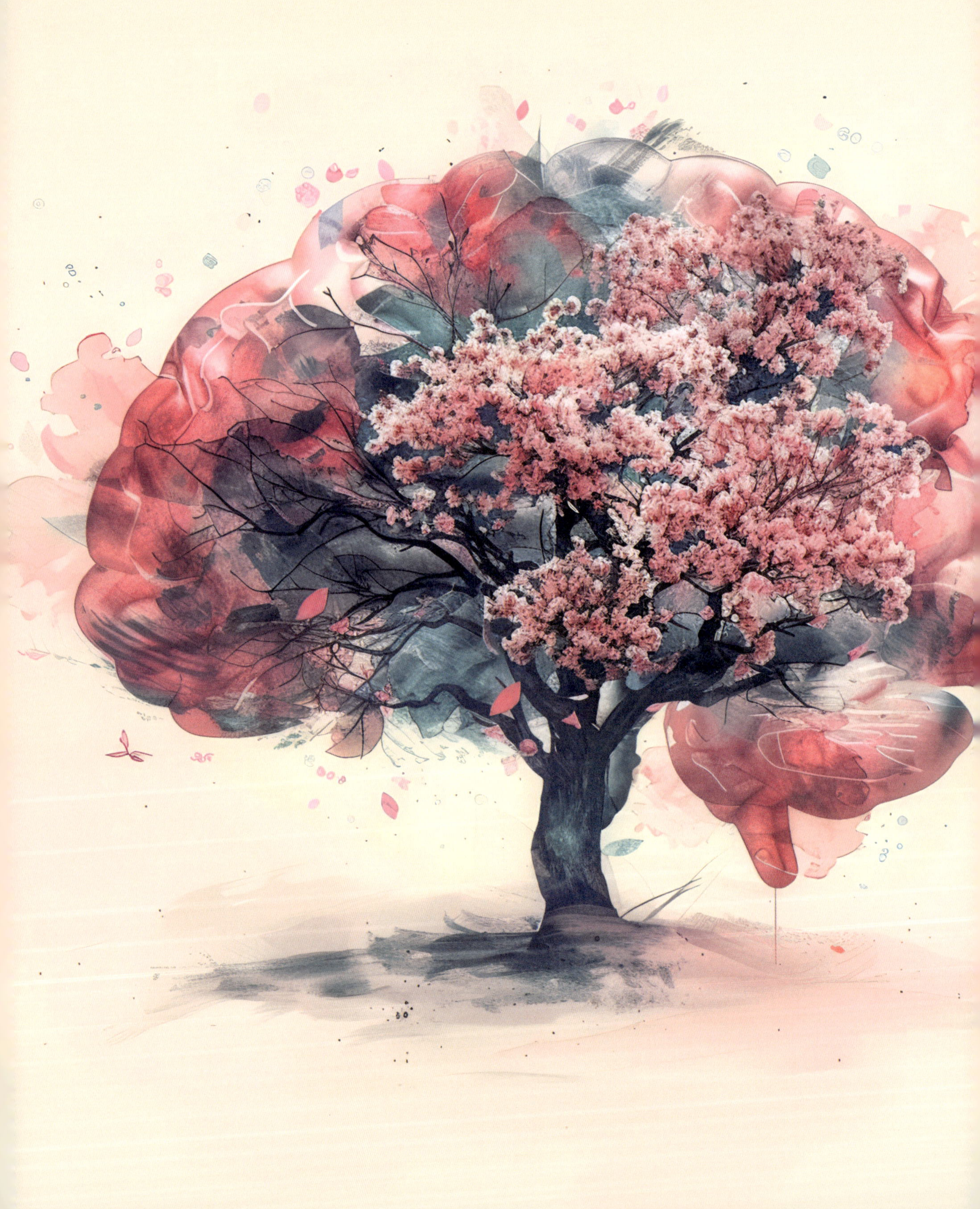

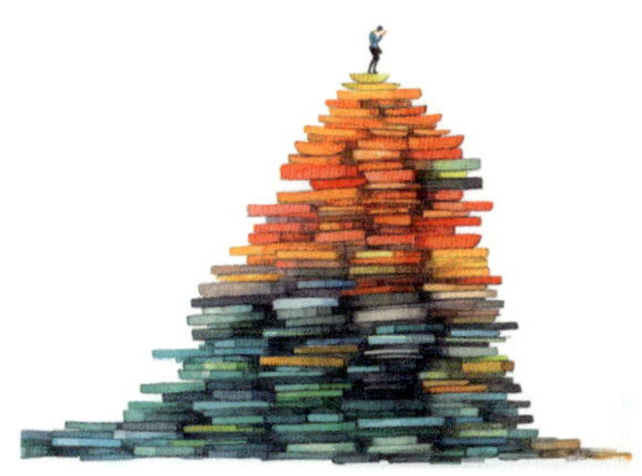
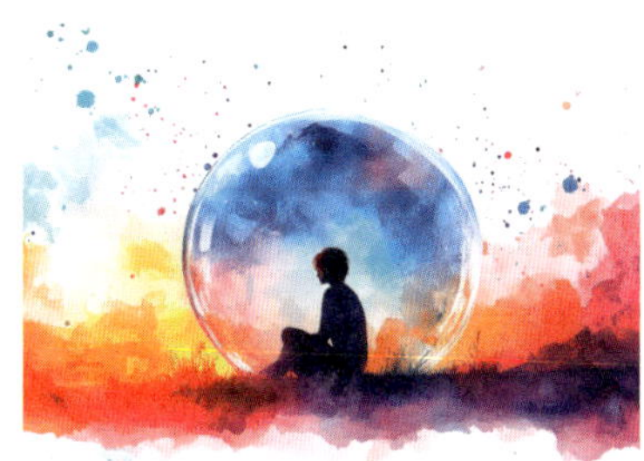
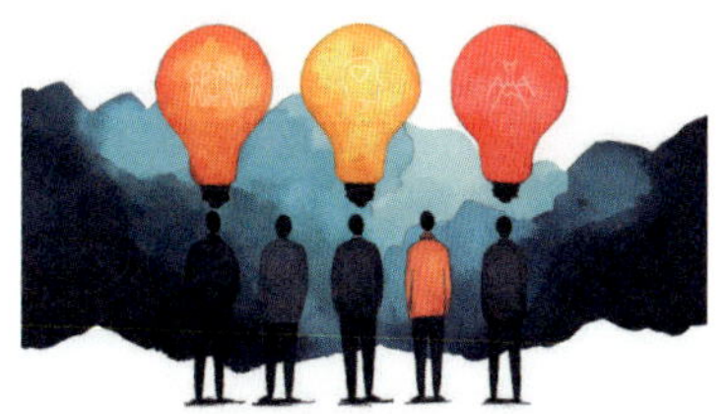

Contents

What Is Anxiety?

Dealing with Anxiety

Solutions

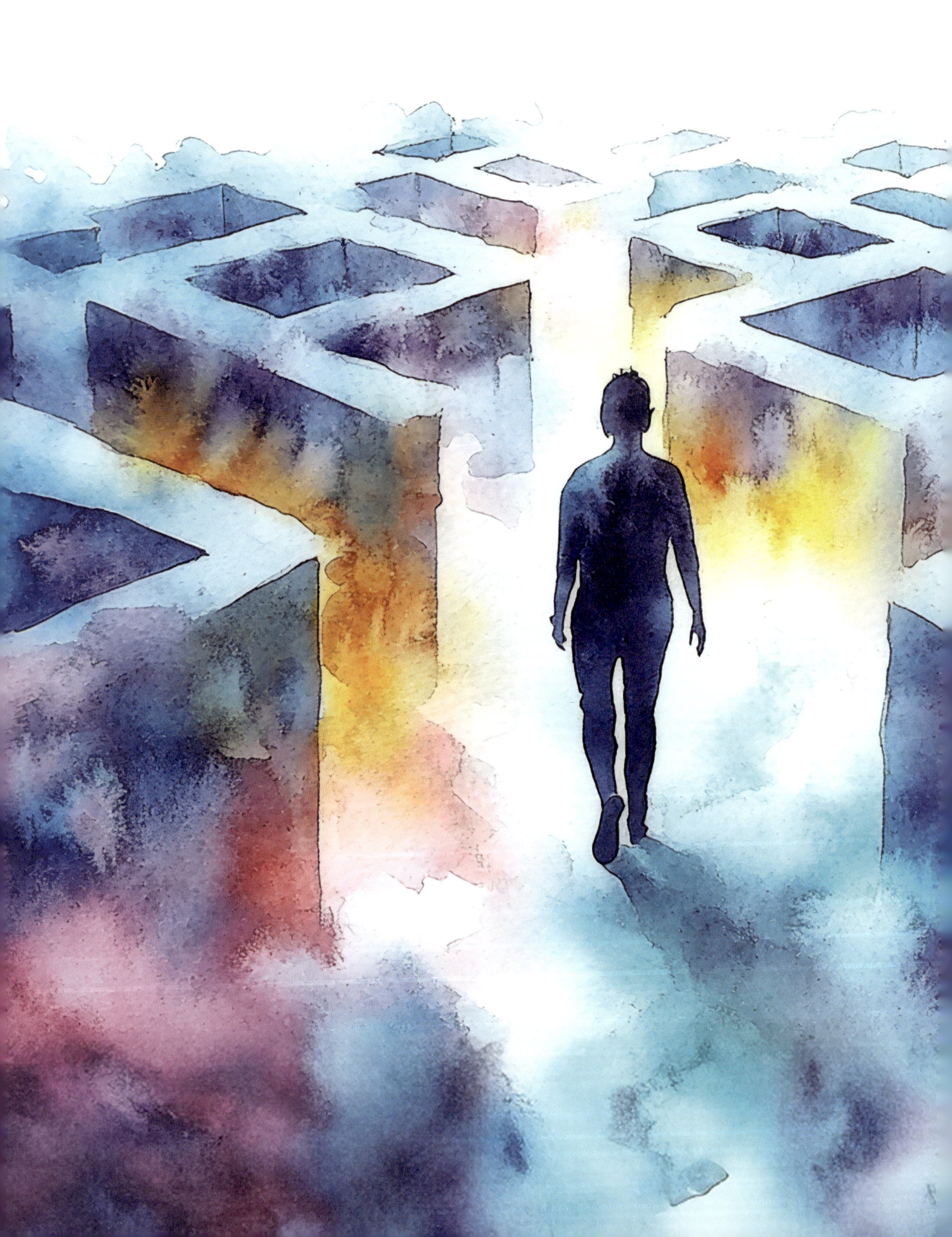

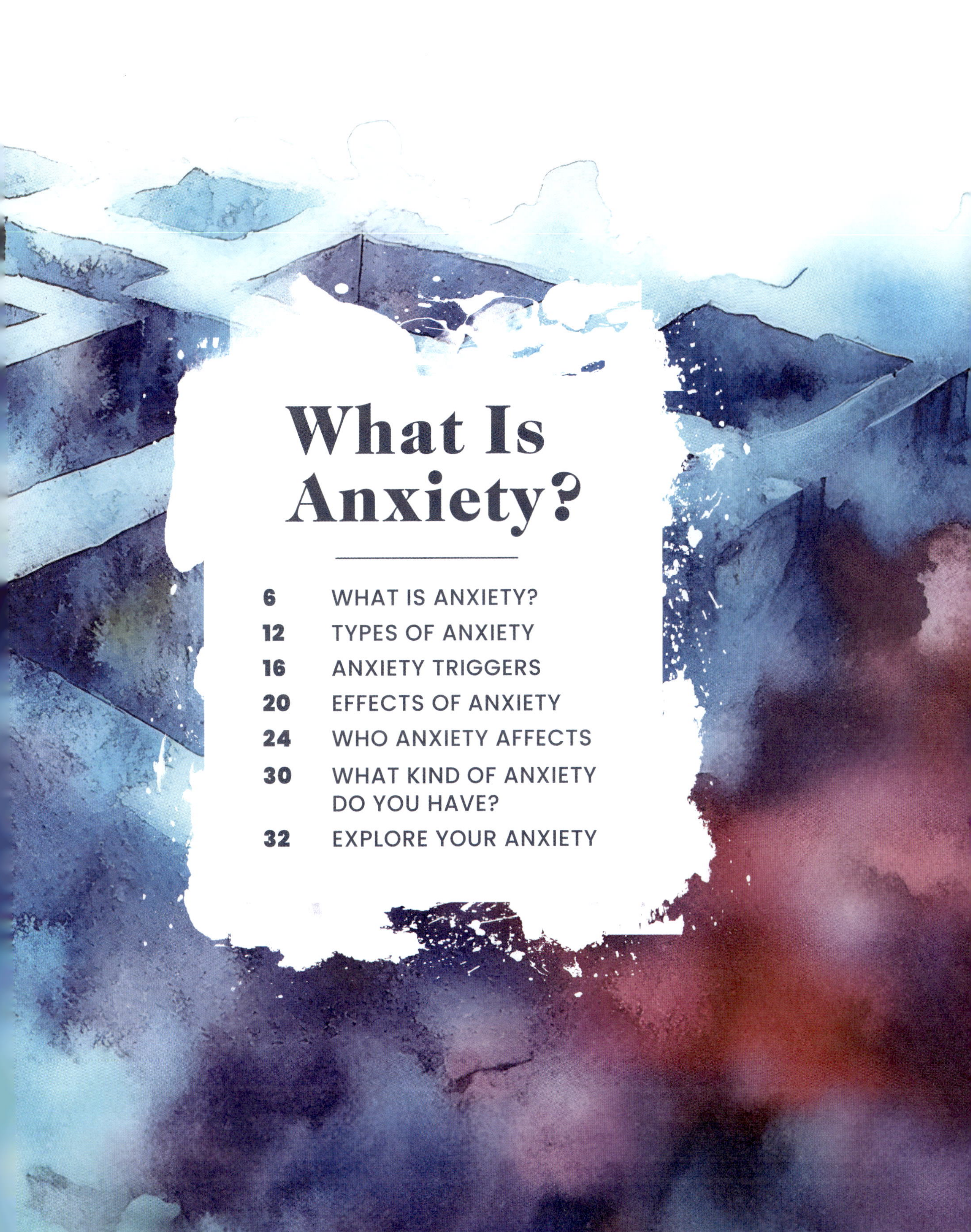

What Is Anxiety?

What Is Anxiety?

UNDERSTAND WHY YOU FEEL ANXIOUS, WHAT'S HAPPENING IN YOUR BRAIN, AND WHO IS MORE VULNERABLE TO IT.

Anxiety is a normal human emotion, triggered in response to stress or perceived danger. Everyone feels anxious from time to time, whether from worrying about a deadline or big presentation, or not being able to get to sleep because your brain is obsessing over things that have happened or might happen. Anxiety can feel like a sensation of general unease or apprehension, or it can be excessive worrying, and it can have both physical and mental effects. Have you ever noticed your heart rate increasing or your palms sweating? Or becoming fixated on what could go wrong with something you're anxious about? This is all normal and part of our built-in "fight-or-flight" response—anxiety puts you in a state of heightened awareness and readiness, prepared to meet the threat head-on.

Anxiety, as an emotion in itself, is not a problem; feeling anxiety from time to time in response to a trigger or stressor is perfectly normal. However, what's not normal is when you're anxious more than usual, when it's impacting on your day-to-day life, and when your level of anxiety is out of proportion to the event or trigger. For example, feeling anxious about getting on stage and speaking in front of a lot of people is something many people experience; getting the same level of anxiety around going to the store, seeing a good friend, or taking a walk is a sign that you're in a state of agitation and dysregulation. This is when feeling a normal level of anxiety tips into having an anxiety disorder, a diagnosable mental health condition where a person feels persistent and intense anxiety.

Anxiety disorder is one of the most common mental health conditions—the World Health Organization (WHO) estimates that 4 percent of the global population currently experience an anxiety disorder, which in 2019 equated to about 301 million people. Anxiety is an umbrella term, and there are many different types, which we'll explore in greater detail. Some people have a more general form of anxiety, where they feel anxious about many aspects of their life; or they may have a more specific type of anxiety linked to a particular trigger. No matter the type of anxiety, the symptoms are the same once triggered, which can include things like heart palpitations, an upset stomach, a tight chest, and shortness of breath.

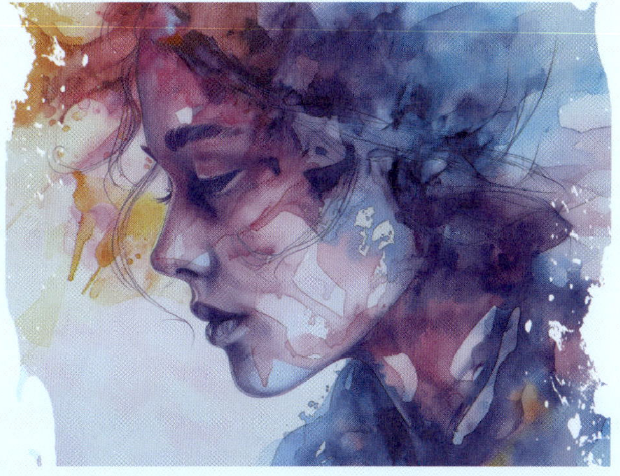

"Your reaction to anxiety is triggered by processes in the brain in reaction to a specific trigger"

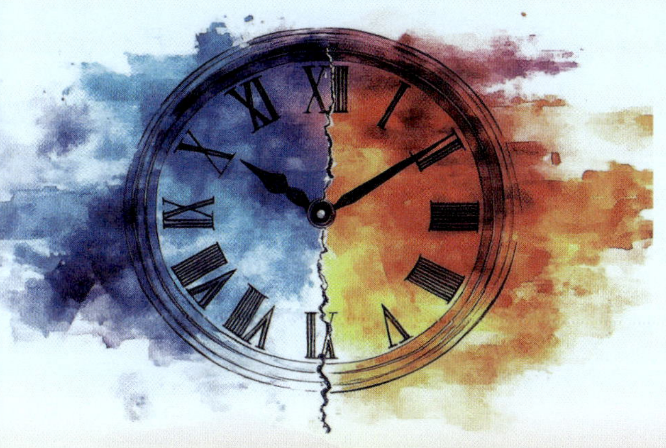

WHAT HAPPENS WHEN YOU'RE ANXIOUS

Your reaction to anxiety is triggered by processes in the brain in reaction to a specific trigger or "threat." First, your amygdala—the area of the brain responsible for processing emotions—identifies something as a threat and sends out

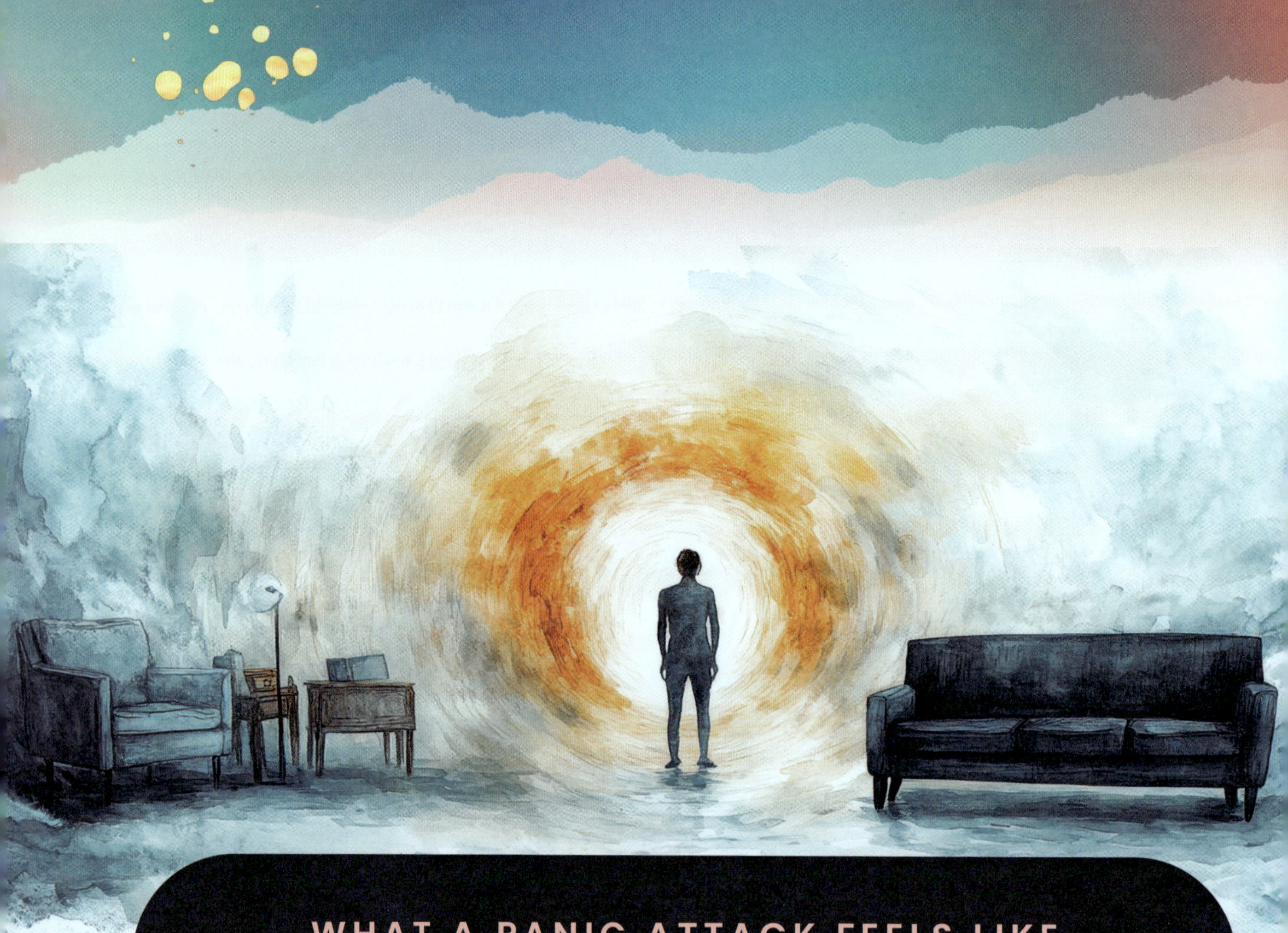

WHAT A PANIC ATTACK FEELS LIKE

Panic is a sudden and overwhelming feeling of fear, and a severe form of anxiety. It can lead to an increase in physical symptoms, such as a rapid heartbeat, shortness of breath, and dizziness. It can be very intense and also lead to irrational behavior. This is called having a "panic attack," and it may be triggered by something specific, but can also come on for no apparent reason. This can lead to people becoming very anxious about having a panic attack, which can then in turn cause a panic attack, creating a constant cycle that can be difficult to get out of. Panic attacks usually last for five to twenty minutes, but they may go on for longer than this.

Panic attacks are not dangerous, but it's important to develop coping strategies, such as breathing deeply, focusing on your inhalation and exhalation, or noticing what you see around you as a way of being in the present moment. Treatment for panic attacks is the same as for anxiety disorder, with talking therapies and cognitive behavioral therapy being very effective, as well as journaling to understand your triggers. Lifestyle modifications can help to manage the underlying anxiety and make panic attacks less likely.

an alarm to the rest of the body to prepare to deal with the problem. Your hypothalamus—responsible for controlling things like your body temperature, heart rate, mood, and hunger—gets this alarm and starts a stress response. This includes raising your blood pressure and heart rate, increasing your breathing rate, and switching your brain into a state of high awareness. The prefrontal cortex is the part of your brain that deals with decision making and reasoning, so it tries to make sense of the threat and put it in context. However, when you're in a state of anxiety, it might not work as it should, being overpowered by the extreme stress response and the overexcited amygdala.

This is all part of the body's natural fight-or-flight system. Your body will prepare for

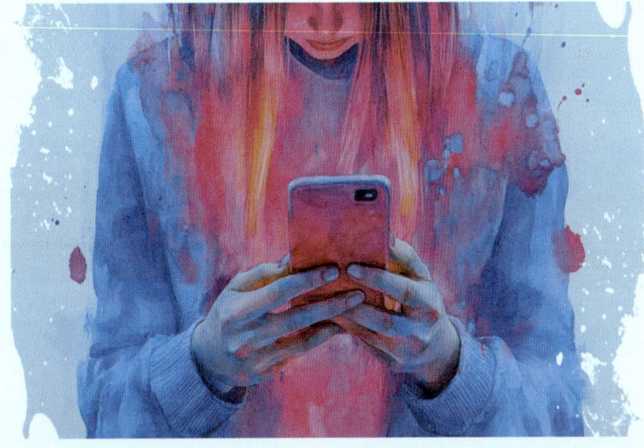

a threat physically as well as mentally. You might feel your muscles go tense, you may get restless and feel a surge of adrenaline—all very useful responses when faced with a real threat. However, when you're in a state of chronic anxiety, having these physical responses regularly and out of proportion to actual threats can lead to longer-term problems. It can impact your immune system, make it difficult to sleep properly, and reduce your capacity for decision-making.

"For some people, anxiety rumbles through their life, whereas for others it is debilitating"

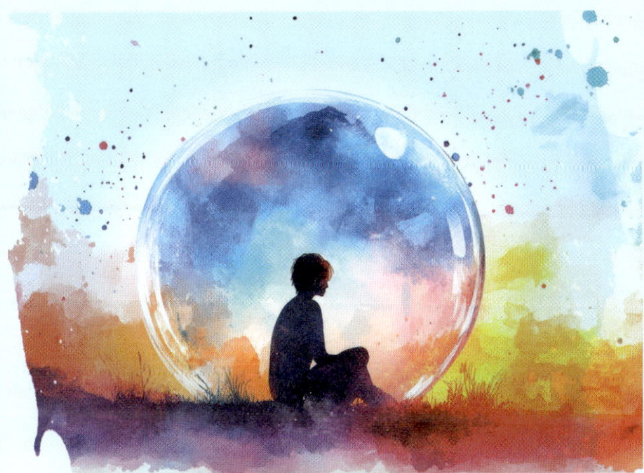

Anxiety disorders also exist on a spectrum; for some people, anxiety rumbles through their life but they're able to go about their daily business, albeit with some difficulties, whereas for others it is debilitating. If you've picked up this book, then anxiety is likely something you struggle with already. The first thing to know is that it's not "just in your head." There is a stigma around anxiety, and it can sometimes be perceived as a weakness. You may also have experienced people telling you to "stop worrying so much" or to "calm down." This can be incredibly frustrating, as it's not possible to simply switch off these emotions. Anxiety is a very real disorder that can have a very big impact on your life and your ability to do things that you normally would. For example, over time anxiety can keep you from engaging in hobbies you enjoy, affect your performance at work, create problems in your relationships with others, and knock your self-esteem.

WHO IS MORE LIKELY TO GET ANXIOUS?

While anyone can have anxiety, there are some traits or vulnerabilities that can make a person more likely to get anxious. Children with anxiety disorders are more likely to have parents who also have anxiety disorders, which could be environmental or biological. Anxiety can run in families, but we don't yet know if this is because of genetics or learned behavior. Women are also twice as likely as men to experience anxiety, according to the Mental Health Foundation.

If you have a lot of stress, this can make you more likely to suffer from anxiety, while stress can also be a result of anxiety. Stress and anxiety overlap in their symptoms, especially as the body reacts in a similar way to fend off the perceived threat. Stress is usually in response to a specific, external situation and is normally a temporary state of being until the external situation resolves itself. Anxiety disorder, however, is persistent and not always related to an external trigger; anxiety can be triggered by things that "might" happen or events in the past.

Those who are prone to overthinking or constantly striving for perfection may also

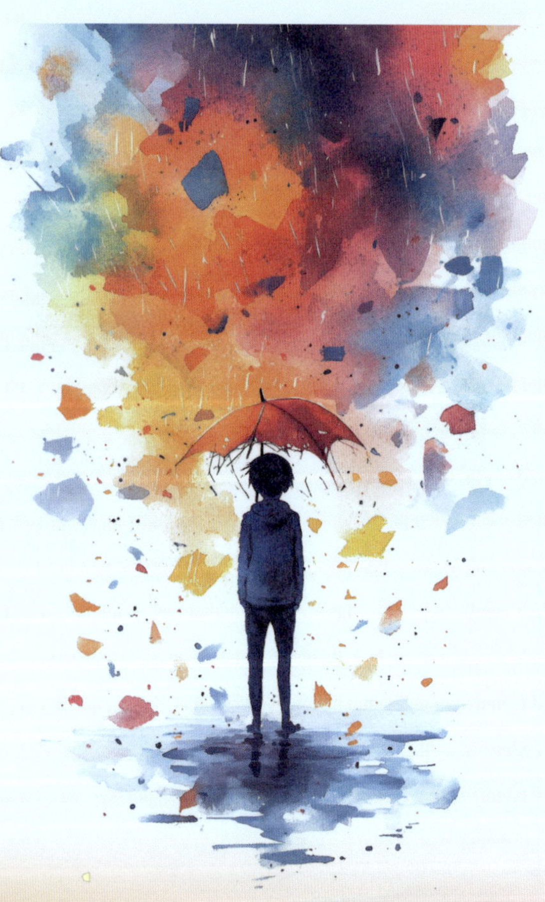

SIGNS & SYMPTOMS

PHYSICAL
- Pounding heart
- Trembling
- Shortness of breath
- Dizziness
- Sweating
- Flushed
- Nausea
- Stomach pains
- Diarrhea
- Restlessness

MENTAL
- Fatigue or tiredness
- Indecisiveness
- Inability to concentrate
- Racing thoughts
- Feeling "on edge"
- Excessive worry
- Poor memory
- Vivid dreams
- Irritability

BEHAVIORAL
- Feeling distressed in social situations
- Obsessive or compulsive behavior
- Avoiding situations
- Responding to overpowering fear

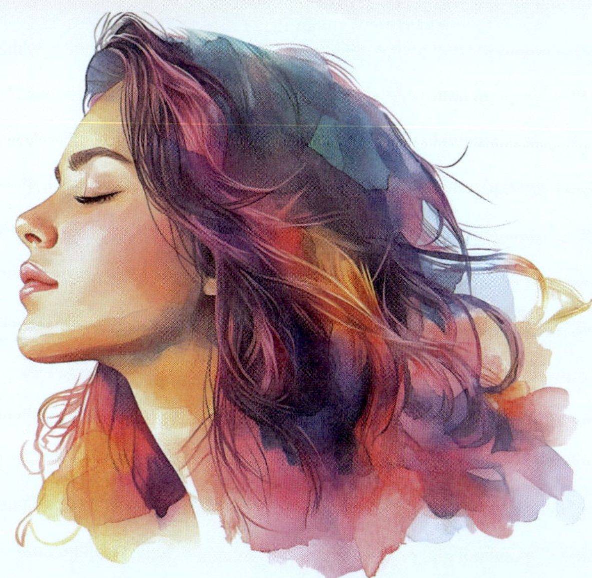

be more likely to suffer from anxiety, as they find it difficult to meet their own impossible expectations, causing excessive worry. Introverted people may be more anxious too, particularly in social scenarios. Social isolation and loneliness can both increase anxiety, as can experiencing trauma, grief, or neglect.

WHAT YOU CAN DO ABOUT ANXIETY

When you're trapped in a state of constant anxiety it can feel like there's no way out, but anxiety is something that can be treated. First, if you haven't already been to a doctor to talk about your anxiety, then this is always recommended, especially if it's having a significant impact on your life. In addition to this, there are certain actions you can take to help manage your anxiety.

In this book we'll walk you through the different techniques, coping mechanisms, and strategies, as well as available treatments, such as talking therapies or medication. This includes things like the lifestyle changes that are most effective in the management of anxiety, and the importance of good nutrition, high-quality sleep, physical activity, having social support, and incorporating mindful movement. We also give you various prompts that help you delve into your triggers, understand your anxiety, and set goals you can work toward. Please don't feel as though you have to work through all the exercises in order. You might find that you're naturally drawn to some more than others, depending on what areas of your anxiety you need to work on most.

"Understanding your anxiety is the first step in gaining control"

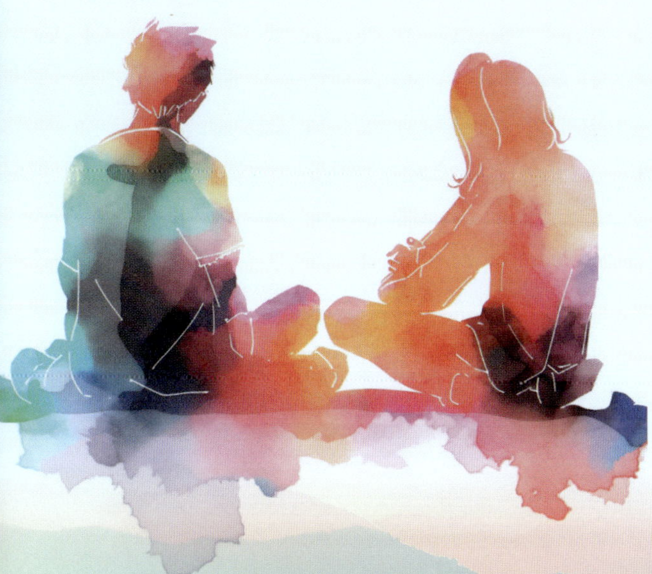

Understanding your anxiety and triggers is the first step in gaining control. The more we learn about it and talk to others about it, the more we can normalize anxiety and find ways to support each other.

Types of Anxiety

FEAR IS A NATURAL AND UNAVOIDABLE PART OF BEING HUMAN, BUT IF IT'S TAKING OVER YOUR LIFE, YOU COULD BE SUFFERING FROM AN ANXIETY DISORDER.

Do you feel constantly burdened with worry? Does fear hold you back from living your life as you'd like to? If the answer is yes, then you could be suffering from an anxiety disorder, a condition in which your natural fear response has become incredibly sensitive and all-consuming, ultimately hampering your quality of life. Dealing with stress at the best of times can be challenging but if you have an anxiety disorder, it can feel overwhelming. These disorders rarely just go away on their own, so it's important to get the right support and treatment so that you can regain control of your mind and life.

Anxiety is normal. It's a natural response that has kept humans alive for millennia; it's that internal alarm that warns us when something isn't right. The problem with anxiety today is that there are more things that can trigger this alarm than ever before. If anxiety stops being temporary and instead hangs around or evolves in intensity, it can transition into a disorder that may get worse over time. Treatment is essential if you want to learn the tools that will help you to cope.

PANIC DISORDER

Panic is the most severe physical form of anxiety, and with this disorder panic attacks usually strike without warning and may happen regularly without treatment. It's no wonder that you might be tempted to avoid certain situations you suspect may trigger an attack, but this only creates a cycle of fear, adding to a foreboding sense of panic. When an attack happens, your way out of it is to focus on your breathing. Keep it slow, deep, and gentle, in through your nose and out through your mouth. Closing your eyes and counting to five for each breath can be a useful distraction, as can repeating to yourself (in your mind) that you are safe. For long-term help, in addition to talking to a medical professional, it can be beneficial to practice self-care (eating, exercising, and sleeping well), relaxation techniques (including mindfulness, which can be achieved by doing a range of hobbies and activities), and stress management.

SOCIAL ANXIETY DISORDER

Formerly referred to as "social phobia," social anxiety impedes your enjoyment of social situations by shrouding you in an overwhelming fear of feeling judged and/or worry of being rejected. More than shyness, social anxiety can take many forms. This can include worrying about talking to strangers—or even friends and family—on the phone or in person, at places you are familiar with, like school or work, or at unfamiliar locations, such as parties. As well as affecting you mentally, this disorder can also create physical signs of stress, such as blushing, sweating, shaking, feeling sick, or panic attacks. When you are experiencing the anxiety, calming your breathing can help. For long-term treatment, consider Cognitive Behavioral Therapy (CBT) counseling (see page 63), while also pursuing regular exercise, self-care, and mindfulness.

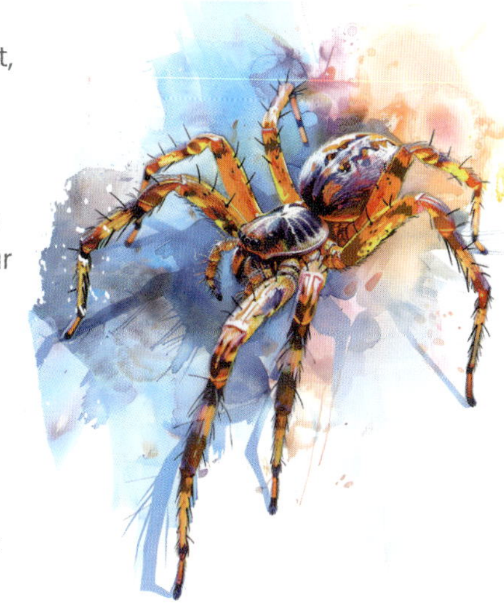

PHOBIAS

Phobias are anxiety disorders. For some people, they may not realize they suffer from one until they experience the thing that creates the fear, while for others, even the thought of something can create anticipatory anxiety. Stronger than a fear, a phobia causes extreme distress and in some cases people alter their lives to avoid coming into contact with the source. It can manifest in physical symptoms, such as rapid heart rate, breathing, sweating, shaking, upset stomach, feeling sick, and panic attacks. Phobias are split into two types: a specific phobia, which is an intense fear of a particular situation, object, animal, or activity (for example dogs, the dentist, flying, heights, etc.), and complex

"Anxiety haunts you by overwhelming you with fears and worry about everything and anything, from day-to-day concerns to dwelling on the past"

phobias, which usually are more deep-rooted in a person's development. The two most common complex phobias include social phobia and agoraphobia, which affects a person's ability to leave home and/or be in open or crowded places. Counseling, CBT, and even hypnotherapy are all valid therapies that sufferers can pursue for getting help with phobias.

GENERALIZED ANXIETY DISORDER (GAD)

If you feel like you're living under a cloud of constant and excessive worry or dread that interferes with your daily life, you may be suffering from GAD. In this form, anxiety haunts you by overwhelming you with fears and worry about everything and anything, from day-to-day concerns to dwelling on events that happened in the past or worrying about things that might happen in the future. The result is that you never feel mentally free to live in the present moment. By ruminating on things that have already happened, asking "What if" or replaying an event where you wish you'd said or done something differently, you're living in the past. Realizing that you can't change the past is a healthy first step to controlling your anxiety. Likewise, overthinking, overplanning, and worrying about how you will deal with things that haven't happened yet is also futile. Trusting yourself to deal with problems as and when they arise is a comforting way to move forward without letting anxiety take hold.

OBSESSIVE-COMPULSIVE DISORDER (OCD)

OCD is a chronic and often long-lasting anxiety disorder where the sufferer has uncontrollable and recurring thoughts and/or behaviors that they are compelled to constantly repeat. OCD affects a person's ability to live a "normal" life because their intrusive thoughts and urges impact every aspect of their daily routine, draining them both mentally and physically. The disorder is thought to manifest in four ways: contamination/cleanliness, doubt/checking, ordering/arranging and unacceptable/taboo thoughts. Unfortunately, OCD won't go away on its own, therefore it's important to seek professional help so that you can learn to acknowledge your obsessions and, in time, become less sensitive to them.

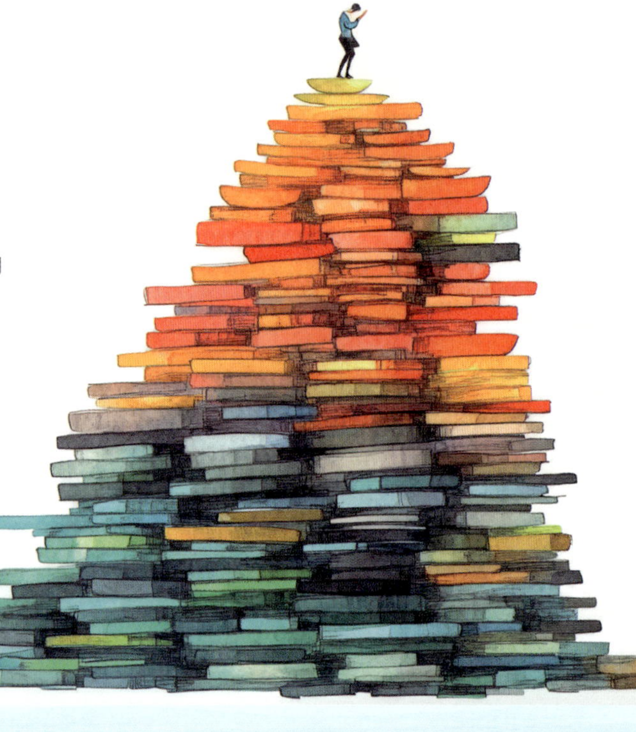

SEPARATION ANXIETY DISORDER

Most parents will experience separation anxiety first-hand when their children start school, and it is a fairly common and natural reaction to being away from their perceived safety net of their family. While most children learn self-coping strategies by the time they are three or four years old, the anxiety disorder can affect adults later in life too. In this form it creates high levels of panic and worry when you aren't with your loved ones. The result is that you can feel withdrawn, intensely sad, lack an appetite, and find it difficult to concentrate or enjoy yourself. You can attempt to deal with this form of anxiety by reminding yourself these feelings are temporary. Keep your brain busy by attempting to identify what triggers these feelings, and try writing them down. Seeing these ideas in black and white can illuminate their irrationality, which can in turn help you to detach yourself from them. The next step is to challenge these negative thoughts and then replace them with positive ones.

POST-TRAUMATIC STRESS DISORDER (PTSD)

PTSD can develop after experiencing a deeply disturbing, distressing, dangerous, and/or damaging situation or event where you experienced an episode of intense fear, helplessness, or stress. PTSD can manifest in a wide range of symptoms, such as flashbacks of the trauma, persistent dwelling, feelings of panic when reminded of the event, or when something triggers the memory and causes you to relive the fear both physically and mentally. You can also experience feelings of detachment and low self-worth, irritability, problems with memory, depression, headaches, mood swings, unusually aggressive behavior, nervousness, sleep disturbances, and many more symptoms. The road to recovery begins with coming to terms with what happened to you. When you feel you are ready, talk to someone you trust to listen without judgment. There is also therapy and/or support groups, and in some cases a health provider may prescribe medication.

"The road to recovery begins with coming to terms with what happened to you. When you're ready, talk to someone you trust"

HEALTH ANXIETY

If you worry a lot about being or becoming ill, you could be suffering from health anxiety. Signs include researching and constantly checking for problems, not trusting doctors, asking people for reassurance, exaggerating an illness, or fabricating one. The trouble with this disorder is that often the anxiety itself creates symptoms of illness (such as nausea, headaches, raised blood pressure and heart rate), creating a cycle that is hard to break. The first step is to distract yourself when you feel yourself starting to worry. For example, when the worry starts, go for a walk, do some yoga, or catch up with a friend. The next step is to take up things you've purposefully avoided, such as socializing, exercise, or a hobby. If self-help doesn't work, then speak to a doctor about CBT.

Anxiety Triggers

LEARNING WHAT CAUSES YOUR ANXIETY IS A HUGE STEP TOWARD UNDERSTANDING AND MANAGING THE DISORDER.

We are all individuals, therefore our experiences of anxiety and what triggers it are unique to each of us. Anxiety disorders are very common, yet discovering what causes anxiety can be a lot more complicated. Often it can come down to a combination of factors, which could include our environment, genetics, or daily habits. What is clear, though, is that some experiences, events, or emotions can trigger the symptoms of anxiety or exacerbate them. Some people experience attacks without first being triggered, while others experience multiple triggers prior to becoming anxious. Given the complex nature of both the human body and anxiety, it's imperative to learn how to identify your own triggers, then you can work on a solution to manage them. Here we examine some common triggers.

HEALTH AND SELF-CARE

Health concerns affect us all, even more so if we experience an upsetting or difficult diagnosis. This stress can often trigger or inflame anxiety and is incredibly powerful due to the personal and immediate feelings it evokes. By being proactive and communicating with your medical health professional you can help to reduce this kind of anxiety. You may even find talking to a therapist useful as they will be trained to help you better understand and manage your diagnosis and emotions surrounding it. Neglecting yourself can also be a trigger, and it's a trait that is surprisingly common among those who experience anxiety. Staying up late, skipping meals, drinking too much alcohol, or not showering regularly are all signs of self-neglect and often an indication of depression, which can also go hand in hand with anxiety.

CAFFEINE

Everyone looks forward to that first coffee of the day. It improves your alertness, increases your energy levels, and puts a smile on your face. You might enjoy it at home when you wake up or on the way to work, but many find this morning necessity actually triggers—and in some cases worsens—their anxiety. For some people it can even induce a panic attack. Because caffeine is a stimulant, it can increase the level of activity in your nervous system. Many products contain caffeine, including favorites such as chocolate, energy drinks, and even some chewing gums. The side effects of caffeine can include increased heart rate and blood pressure, insomnia, heart palpitations and, of course, anxiety. By substituting your caffeinated drinks for decaf options and cutting back on your caffeine intake, you may well notice a difference in your body.

FINANCES

In the current climate there are so many people who have financial worries. These money concerns can trigger anxiety because in our minds we associate money with survival. Having money can often provide us with a sense of security and therefore safety, so it stands to reason that when people have fears about their financial situation, they may start to worry about their safety. Be it fretting about job security, a lack of savings, mounting bills, debt, identity theft, or sudden unexpected outgoings, worrying about money can often lead to disrupted sleep patterns, and sometimes even simple tasks like opening envelopes or attending appointments can trigger feelings of panic and anxiety. Financial worries can also have a huge impact on a person's relationships and social life, which can, in turn, leave them feeling isolated or lonely.

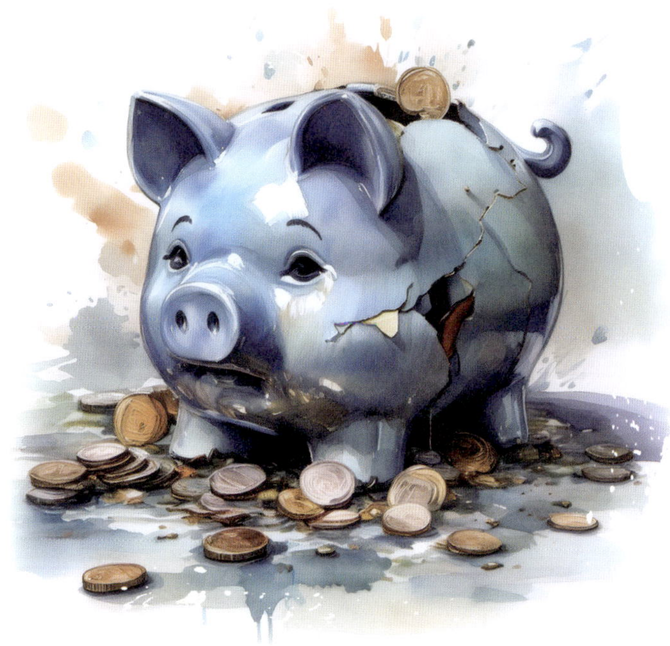

UNHEALTHY RELATIONSHIP WITH FOOD

Our relationship with food is hugely important to both our body and mind, and what we do or don't consume can greatly affect our mood. Being "hangry" (hungry to the point of feeling angry and frustrated) is just one example of how our diet can dictate our mood. When we are hungry, our stomachs rumble and our hands sometimes tremble. This can be down to a drop in our blood sugar levels, and it is also a trigger for anxiety. Balanced meals not only provide us with important nutrients and vitamins but also with the energy our bodies need to steer us through the day. A healthy, well-balanced diet can help prevent low blood sugar, in addition to staving off negative feelings of agitation, anxiety, and nervousness.

NEGATIVE THOUGHTS

One of the biggest triggers for anxiety is the way in which we think and speak to ourselves. This can leave us feeling frustrated and upset, which subsequently fuels anxiety. The mind controls a great deal of the body, which is why when we experience negative thoughts, particularly about ourselves, we increase the chances of triggering an episode. For example, just thinking "I am not good enough" or "No one understands me" is enough to start a negative spiral. However, there is a way to combat negativity. Trying to replace negative thoughts with more positive and realistic ones is a helpful method, as is keeping a diary to track your thoughts—in time this could reveal a pattern. You may also find working with a therapist productive when it comes to learning how to refocus your language and internal voice.

PRIVATE TRIGGERS

Your own personal triggers are unique and often private to you. People who experience PTSD often have anxiety brought on by environmental triggers, but some can be caused by a particular place, a song, or even a smell that takes someone back to a place in their mind that causes a reaction. Remember there is no right or wrong way to experience anxiety. You are not strange for refusing to pick up the phone to a number you don't recognize or for feeling nervous in a restaurant when it comes to ordering food. Many people worry about being in an unknown location and not being able to find the bathroom or exit. Sometimes these personal triggers may even be experienced

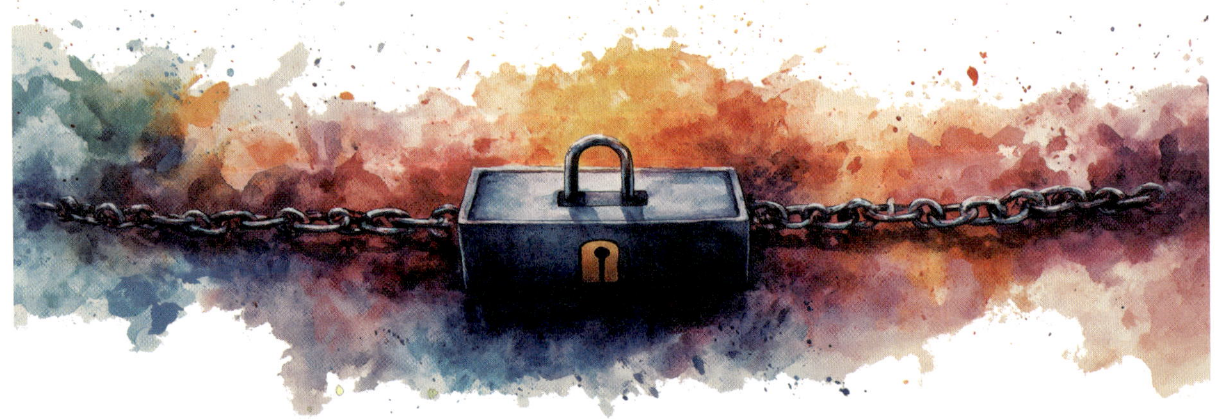

subconsciously, making them even more difficult to identify. With help from a mental health specialist, you can learn not only how to identify them, but also how to overcome them.

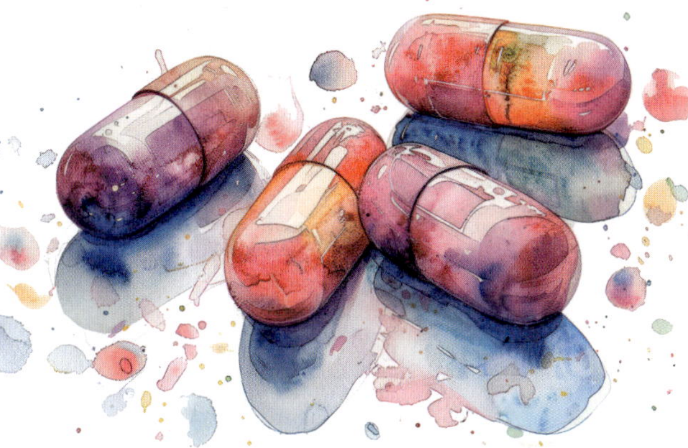

MEDICATION

Studies show that many over-the-counter medications and prescriptions, including birth-control tablets, weight-loss pills, and cough medicine, can actually trigger anxiety. This is due to the ingredients in them, which can leave you feeling unwell or uneasy and have the potential to ignite a chain reaction that may cause further symptoms. Be sure to read all of the information provided with your medications to see what side effects you might experience and discuss with your doctor. Where possible, see if you can find an alternative therapy or medication that doesn't worsen your symptoms or trigger your anxiety.

YOUR SAFE SPACE

Your home and space is often a reflection of you, and having a messy home environment can cause an individual with anxiety a great deal of stress. Your mental "to-do list" can be vast, and having lots of jobs on it, such as cleaning, can be a trigger. This can then result in a reduced ability to focus, increased levels of stress, and insomnia. Keeping your home as orderly as possible is a proven way to diminish anxiety. Try writing a physical to-do list to help remove the stress from your mind by getting it down on paper.

RELATIONSHIPS

Sometimes the fear of confrontation can render a person with anxiety completely mute. Not being able to articulate what we really want to say can cause ineffective communication, even with loved ones. A person's upbringing can also trigger episodes. From not feeling heard to physical or mental abuse, past experiences can play a huge part when it comes to anxiety. The modern world is not particularly conducive to remaining calm, given that many people spend a lot of time on social media comparing themselves to others. We also expose ourselves by commenting on other people's posts, risking negative or unkind feedback. Taking time to enjoy the world outside is essential for our mental and physical well-being, as are spells away from screens, negative news, and upsetting images.

WORK AND SOCIAL INTERACTIONS

Anxiety brought on by work and social interactions is common. Making a presentation or speaking to a room full of people can be a trigger. Talking with a doctor or therapist can help in working out ways to make you feel more comfortable in these settings. Interacting with good friends who make you feel comfortable will also help, as will positive reinforcements from colleagues and family. Surrounding yourself with positive influences can also make you feel more confident.

Effects of Anxiety

ANXIETY CAN AFFECT YOU MENTALLY, PHYSICALLY, AND EMOTIONALLY, IMPACTING YOUR ACTIONS AND BEHAVIOR.

When you're anxious, you're more than just worried about something. Anxiety is an emotion that can have a huge effect on your whole body. You might not be aware of all the symptoms of anxiety, but by learning what they are, you may discover you experience more of them than you thought. Learning to recognize these signs early means you can implement coping strategies before the symptoms get more intense.

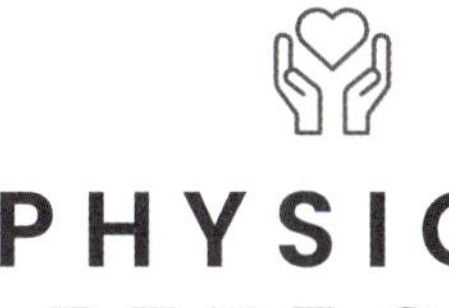

PHYSICAL EFFECTS

Because anxiety triggers certain processes in the brain, various parts of your body react to the perceived "threats." One of the most common physical symptoms is an increase in heart rate or heart palpitations, which is when your heartbeat feels more rapid or irregular than usual. Some people even feel chest pain—this is something that should never be ignored, and if you get chest pain often, you should get it checked out by a doctor to ensure it is a symptom of anxiety and nothing more.

You might also find that your breathing is more rapid or that it's harder to take a full breath, which is why breathing exercises can be so effective; when you get your breathing back under control, it can help you to feel calmer overall. Because your breathing is more rapid or shorter than usual, you might also notice that you feel a little dizzy or lightheaded. Some people get pins and needles or other tingling sensations, as their nervous system is under stress. With the racing heartbeat and irregular breathing, you might also find that you start to sweat more than normal or have tremors in your limbs.

Many people with anxiety also suffer from gastrointestinal symptoms, such as an upset stomach leading to diarrhea, or constipation and bloating. You may also feel nauseous or notice a jittery sensation in your stomach.

Anxiety can mean you hold a lot of tension in the body, and you may notice this—along with pain—in areas like your neck, shoulders, and back. When the symptoms are short-lived, you can get them back under control using relaxation techniques, but if your anxiety is long term, these symptoms can lead to other physical health problems, such as heart conditions or stomach ulcers.

"Anxiety can mean you hold a lot of tension in the body, along with pain in your neck..."

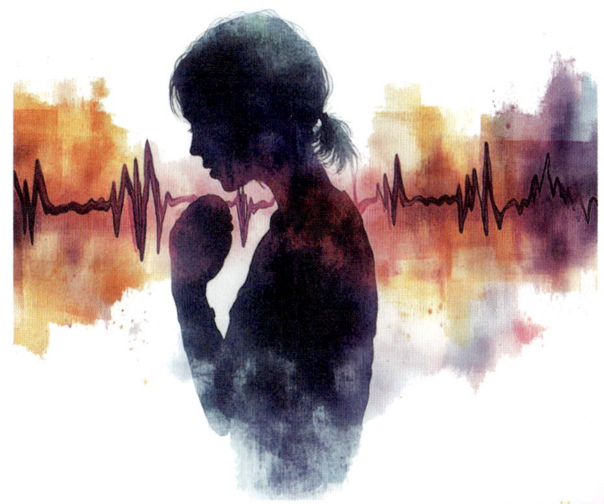

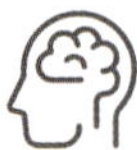

MENTAL EFFECTS

Anxiety is a mental health condition, which means it has many mental and emotional symptoms alongside the physical symptoms. These can range in severity, and in some people the mental symptoms can be truly debilitating. The most common mental symptom is excessive worry and fear. Many people have a persistent feeling of apprehension or dread, a sense that something bad is going to happen, and a focus on the worst possible outcome. There is a tendency to dwell on these negative thoughts, and they can often intrude at unhelpful times. It can be hard to catch and recognize these thoughts, and this pattern of negative thinking can prevent you from going about your normal day-to-day life. It is mentally exhausting to spend so much time worrying, but it is difficult to stop. The techniques in this book will help you learn how to control and manage this.

Because the brain is so busy processing this worry, it can become hard to concentrate and focus on other tasks. This can impact everything from your ability to study or work, to being able to sit and enjoy something on television or read a book. It can also impact your ability to make decisions, especially if you're worried about making a wrong decision, and it can also affect your short-term memory as it can be hard to take new information in. When you're in this state of anxiety, you'll also find it harder to relax as you feel alert to any potential threats, and your brain may feel constantly busy. This can then make it difficult to sleep.

When you're tired and overwhelmed, it can make you more irritable and you may find it harder to stay calm. You may have mood swings, sometimes feeling overly tearful or overwhelmed, and other times feeling frustrated and angry. This can then make it harder to keep your emotions under control. In worst-case scenarios, if severe anxiety is not caught and treated, it can even lead to disconnection from your body and from reality.

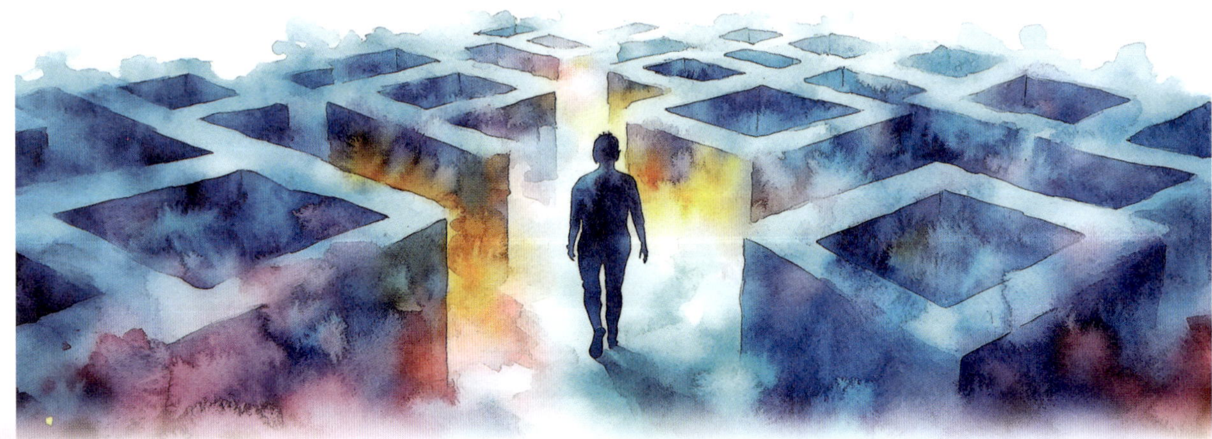

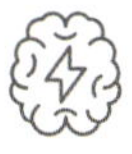

BEHAVIOR AND ACTIONS

These physical and mental symptoms of anxiety can influence your behavior and actions. It's not uncommon to start avoiding situations or activities that trigger your anxiety, even if it's something you've always enjoyed. Sometimes it can just feel easier not to do something than it does to work through your anxiety and figure out a way to cope. Unfortunately, if you start a pattern of avoidance, your brain will always want to take the easy way out and you may find you start avoiding more and more situations. This can then make it more difficult to start doing things again without some support.

Along with avoidance, you may also find yourself beginning to withdraw socially—not responding to friends and family when they reach out. This might be because you are anxious about seeing them, because you think they may judge you for your anxiety, or because you don't want to explain why you're avoiding their messages or invitations. We know how important social support is in the treatment of anxiety, and we have some advice later in this book to help you build a support network and speak to trusted friends.

"It's not uncommon to start avoiding situations that trigger your anxiety"

When you have anxiety, you may adopt other unhelpful behaviors as a way of coping. Some people lose their appetite and find it hard to stick to a routine of regular meals; other people find they eat more because they use food as an emotional crutch to help them feel better, in the same way some people turn to things like alcohol, smoking, or recreational drugs to try to stave off the anxiety they're feeling. The restlessness and irritability can also lead to habits such as nail biting, skin picking, teeth grinding, and pacing back and forth.

How many of the symptoms we've outlined here do you recognize in yourself? Acknowledging these symptoms as part of your anxiety is the first step in learning how to control them.

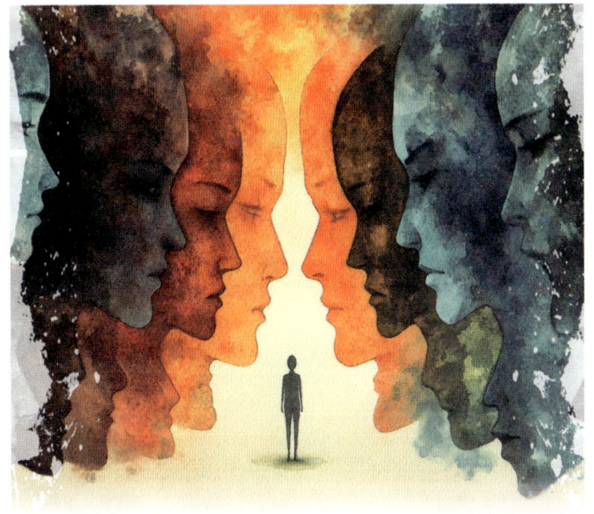

Who Anxiety Affects

NO MATTER WHO YOU ARE, ANXIETY CAN STRIKE. HERE ARE SOME OF THE WAYS IT CAN AFFECT DIFFERENT PEOPLE.

We are all different, and we all respond to stress and worries in our own unique ways. When worries and stresses become too much, however, they might affect our everyday lives, impact on our physical and emotional health, and become difficult to manage. Anyone can be vulnerable to anxiety disorders, no matter their age, gender identity, or race. But sometimes anxiety can have certain triggers and effects, or present itself differently, depending on who you are and what your individual life experience has been.

Learning about how anxiety affects different people isn't just useful for understanding our own anxiety journey, though. Being aware of how anxiety can impact someone else can enable us to empathize with them as well as help us recognize symptoms in ourselves. But remember, anxiety can be different for everyone, and this is just a guide.

ANXIETY ACROSS SOCIETY

Anxiety may feel different for everyone, but the list of possible symptoms is broadly the same, no matter your gender or race. However, some groups disproportionately suffer with anxiety; for example, women are more likely to be diagnosed with anxiety than men (although it should be noted that this may be due to many factors, which may include underdiagnosis in men).

Trans and non-binary people also disproportionately struggle with mental health difficulties compared to cisgender people. People coming to terms with a gender identity different to the gender assigned at birth face unique barriers in society—and these can understandably take a toll on mental health. Helplines and organizations such as the Trevor Project and the National Alliance on Mental Illness provide specific support for trans and non-binary people who are suffering with anxiety or other mental health problems.

Experiencing racism can also have a profound impact on mental health, and is considered a trigger for anxiety. A recent study by mental health charity Mind also found that one in three people from marginalized communities had encountered discrimination or judgment when seeking support for their mental health.

It is important to be mindful of the powerful link between life experience and mental health. No matter what your background or situation, if anxiety symptoms are affecting your daily life, seek help from a doctor, relevant support organization, or a mental health organization or charity.

"Anyone can be vulnerable to anxiety disorders, no matter their age, gender identity, or race"

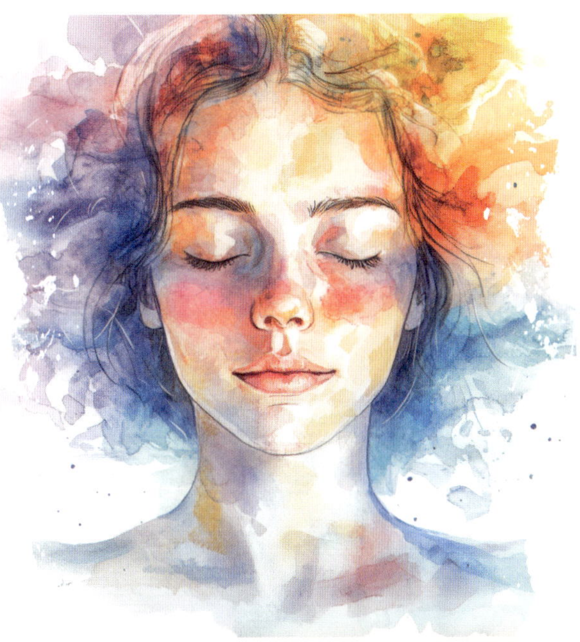

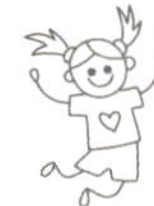

ANXIETY IN CHILDREN

Children can't always communicate their feelings articulately, and can't always understand their emotions. As parents, caregivers, or adults working with children, it can therefore be useful to know the common signs of anxiety disorders in children.

It's important to state that being anxious from time to time is normal for many children, as it is for adults. But when anxious feelings are affecting their daily life, it may be time to seek out professional advice.

Signs of an anxiety disorder to look out for in a child include:

- Not eating well
- Difficulty sleeping, bad dreams
- Inability to concentrate
- Being irritable or frequently angry
- Expressing constant worries or negative thoughts
- Being extra clingy or tearful

Anxious children might also complain of a stomachache or feeling unwell, or need to use the toilet often.

Children can feel anxious about school, friends, family, the news, or any number of stresses they are struggling to deal with. When you are in a calm, quiet, and safe environment, ask them how they are feeling, if they have any worries—and how that makes them feel, emotionally and physically.

A different type of anxiety—separation anxiety—is a normal part of development for very young children, between six months and three years old. This happens as the child learns more about their world and begins to understand their reliance on caregivers.

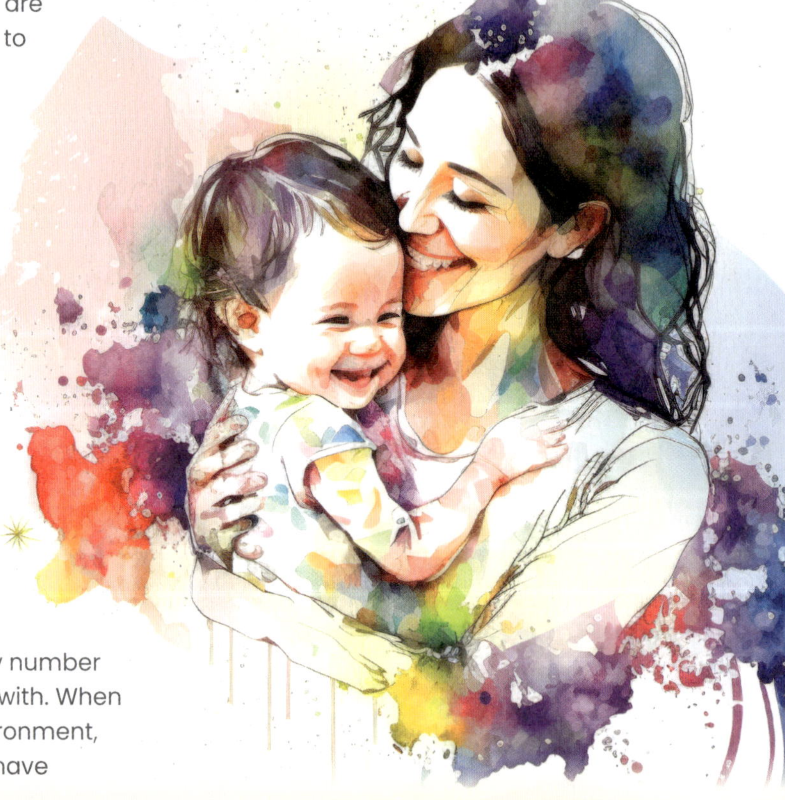

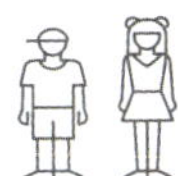

TEENAGE ANXIETY

The teenage years are difficult for even the most resilient of children, bringing new concerns alongside physical changes.

School can be a trigger for anxiety in teenagers, with pressure often placed on their achievements as they move toward higher education or the working world. It's important to let them know that although hard work is important, they are supported and have options if things don't go to plan.

Social pressures can also weigh on teenagers, whether that's among peers in person, or online.

Watching the news and thinking about the future can be daunting, especially for teenagers coming to terms with their place in an uncertain world.

Make sure to watch for any changes in behavior, such as communicating fears and worries more often; avoiding school or regular activities they once enjoyed; having trouble sleeping; and complaining of headaches, tiredness, or stomachache. If you're worried about these symptoms, speak to your teenager and your doctor about seeking help.

"Watching the news and thinking about the future can be daunting, especially for teenagers coming to terms with their place in an uncertain world"

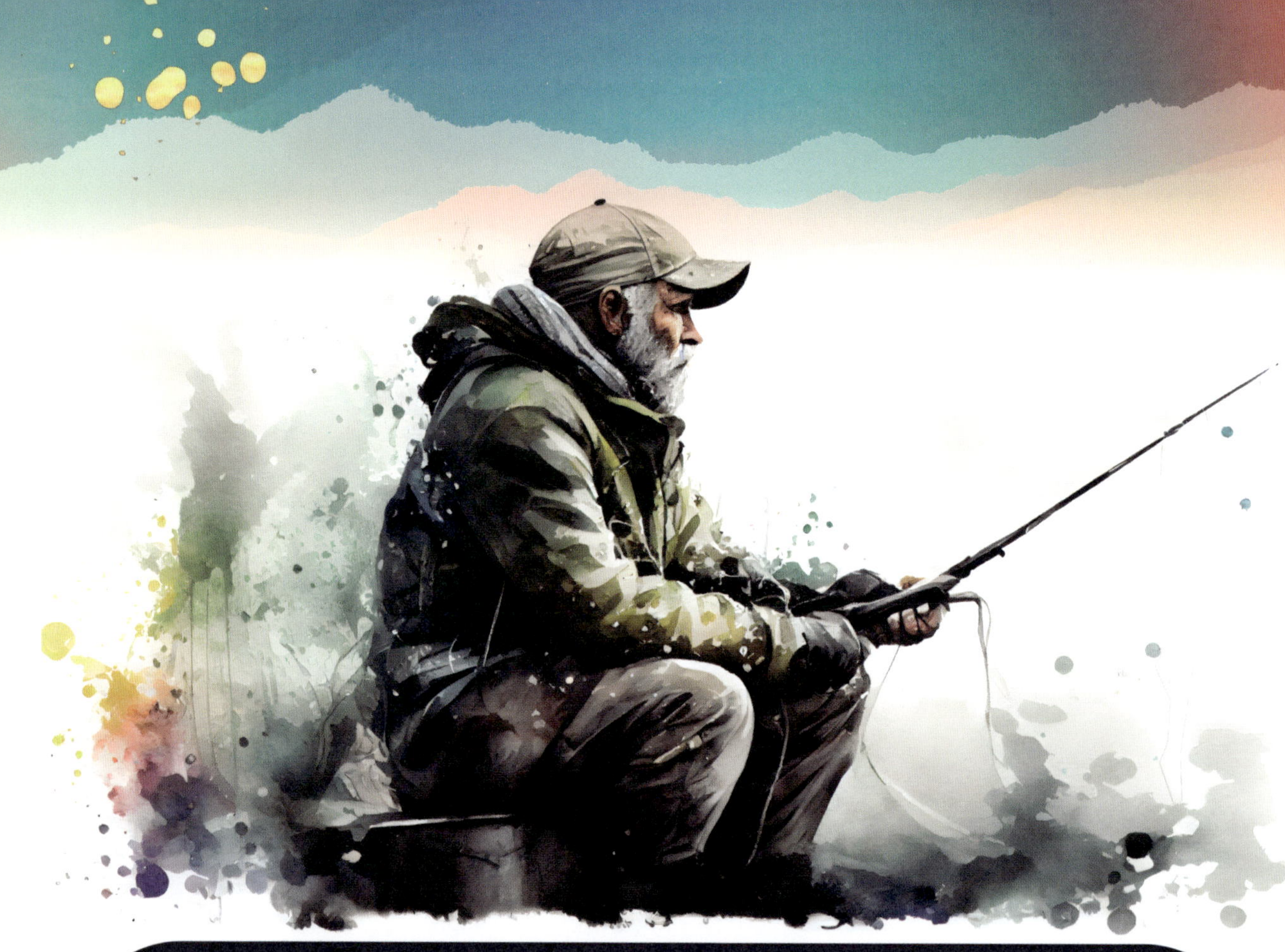

ENCOURAGING MEN TO SEEK HELP

Data has shown that men are less likely to seek help for their mental health than women. This may be due to "traditional" views of masculinity, in which men were not encouraged to discuss their emotions. Men may have felt that fear or embarrassment were also barriers to seeking help, perhaps as a result of these historic perceptions of masculinity.

In order to help break down these boundaries, look out for signs of anxiety in men and encourage discussing feelings and worries openly. In addition to the most common anxiety symptoms, men may also immerse themselves further into work or hobbies as an escape, take more risks, or experience physical symptoms such as stomach issues or headaches. People of any gender or background may have these symptoms, but they may also be subtler ways of men trying to cope with anxiety.

If you suspect someone you know is suffering, approach the subject in a calm and open way, asking about their feelings. You could also express your concern. It may not be received well—just make sure they know you are there to offer support. And if you are a man who is suffering, don't delay seeking help from a doctor.

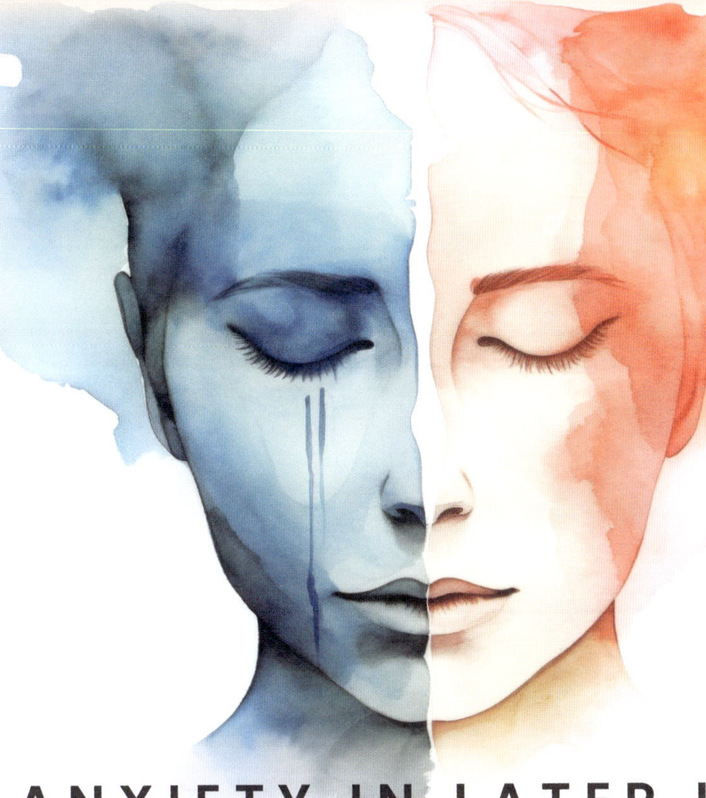

AGE AND WORRY
Anxiety is the most common type of mental health disorder in older adults, according to the Anxiety and Depression Association of America.

ANXIETY IN LATER LIFE

Much like anxiety in younger people, an anxiety disorder in later years can cause a feeling of constantly being "on edge," feeling sick, an inability to control worries, and irritability. When these symptoms linger and make everyday life more difficult, it's time to consult a doctor and seek treatment. There won't be any judgment, and it's common for people of all ages, including older adults, to feel this way at times.

Later life brings with it a host of potential concerns that can weigh on the mind, including financial worries, bereavement, caring for loved ones, moving house, and coping with retirement, among many others. If there are significant changes happening in your life, or to somebody close to you, stay in touch with close friends and family and talk about the effects of these changes regularly if you can. Older people need and deserve support through these momentous life changes, just as younger people do.

Anxiety can also be triggered by recurring events such as the changing seasons or chronic health problems. If you or a loved one has suffered with anxiety in the past, watch out for triggers and stay alert to symptoms of returning anxiety. Don't be afraid to seek help if you feel anxiety is becoming unmanageable.

What Kind of Anxiety Do You Have?

IDENTIFY THE AREAS IN YOUR LIFE THAT GIVE YOU THE MOST ANXIETY.

There are many different types of anxiety, which are broadly categorized by the scenarios or thoughts that trigger a reaction. Here we explore the most common types of anxiety, but you may find that you have a mix of all/some of them. There are other types of anxiety not covered, such as phobias and panic disorder. This is not intended to be a diagnostic tool, but it can help you to identify what makes you feel most anxious so you can find a coping mechanism. For each question, choose the answer that best reflects how you feel most of the time.

ANXIETY SCALE Use this scale to see whether or not to seek help.

MINIMAL
Minimal effects of anxiety will have very few physical symptoms, if any at all. You'll have small feelings of worry but will be able to get things done and focus on tasks.

MILD
At this level you may get stomachaches and feel muscle tension. Your sleep and concentration may be affected and you'll feel anxious throughout the day, but not all day.

MODERATE
Moderate levels of anxiety might mean that you are anxious for the majority of the day—you might be feeling panicky, tired, and getting headaches. It's likely that you'll experience changes in your sleep, appetite, and ability to concentrate.

SEVERE
Severe anxiety will mean that you are feeling anxious all day. You might experience shortness of breath, chest tightness, or digestive issues. You might feel overwhelmed and want to isolate yourself, as well as being unable to focus.

DEBILITATING
Debilitating levels of anxiety will mean that you'll have severe symptoms all day. You won't be able to function and will be experiencing severe physical symptoms. You might be having meltdowns, feel paralyzed, and unable to continue.

QUIZ

When I'm trying to get to sleep at night, I mostly:

A Worry about what went wrong today or could go wrong tomorrow

B Replay conversations or social interactions in my head

C Worry about a health problem or symptom that's bothering me

D Any or all of the above

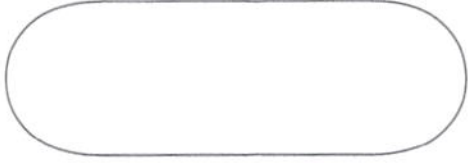

When I'm invited to a social event, my initial reaction is to:

A Worry about the logistics, what could go wrong, and how to fit it in

B Fixate on what I might say wrong or how to converse to the people who are there

C Be concerned that I could get ill before the event, or even catch something there

D Find it all too overwhelming and want to decline the invitation

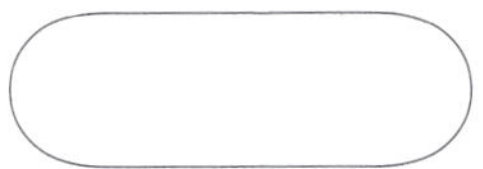

When I'm feeling most anxious, I'm most likely dwelling on:

A What I have to do, how I'm going to do it, and what decisions I have to make

B How people see me and what they think about me

C My body and how it's feeling, and what symptoms I might have

D Any or all of the above

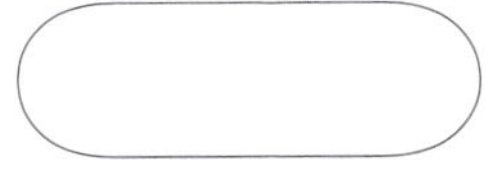

The situation that would cause me the most anxiety would be:

A Making an error or missing a deadline at work

B Having to stand up and give a speech in front of people

C Experiencing an unexplained ache or pain

D Any or all of the above

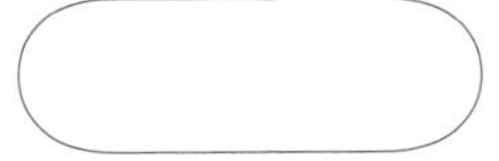

When something goes wrong, my initial thought is:

A "This messes up everything; how will I cope?"

B "What will people think when they find out?"

C "Is this a sign that there is something wrong with me?"

D "It's too overwhelming"

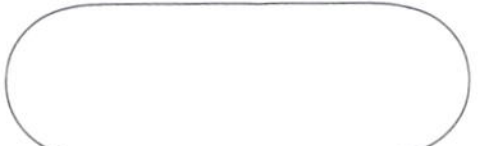

MOSTLY As

General Anxiety—you worry about lots of different things in your daily life, including dwelling on the past and what might happen in the future.

MOSTLY Bs

Social Anxiety—you have a fear of social situations and the way that others perceive you, worrying that you might say the wrong thing, act the wrong way, or just generally feel judged.

MOSTLY Cs

Health Anxiety—you spend a lot of time worrying that you're already ill or going to get ill, and constantly check your body for new symptoms or health concerns.

MOSTLY Ds

Mixed Anxiety—you identify with aspects of all of the above. Many people have different types of anxiety at the same time that overlap.

CONCLUSION

No matter the result, the exercises and advice in this book can help you manage your anxiety. If you're struggling, and it's really impacting your normal day-to-day life, make an appointment to see your doctor.

Explore Your Anxiety

UNDERSTANDING THE CAUSE OF YOUR ANXIETY WILL HELP YOU FIND SOLUTIONS.

Now that you have learned all about what anxiety is, you can take a look at how you deal with it. Over the following pages, spend some time thinking about what makes you anxious. Make a list of your anxieties, write down what type of anxiety you have, and what symptoms you have. Think about different types of situations where you feel anxious and how you react to stress. How does anxiety affect you? What do you think your triggers are? Write these down. Then come back to these pages when you've read through the other sections of the book and think about what you can do to help you cope. Think about your successes, challenges, and lessons learned, and consider any patterns you might have noticed, areas you still need to work on, and what tools have been effective for you.

Everyone will have started in different places. Some might have had a bit of daily anxiety they wanted to get on top of, while others might have struggled with more severe anxiety for a long time. It's a very individual journey that's probably had many ups and downs.

The goal of a book like this isn't to get rid of anxiety completely; it's not a "cure." It's been designed to help you learn to manage anxiety and feel more in control of it—rather than letting anxiety have control over you. Hopefully, it'll help you get into some good habits, whether that's through lifestyle tweaks or journaling, which you can continue going forward.

When you've finished reading through the book, take a moment to reflect on what's changed. What does your life look like now in comparison to how it was when you started reading this book? Do you feel more relaxed? Have you managed to do activities you wouldn't have been able to before? Have you opened up to anyone about the way you're feeling? Have you started a treatment plan? These are all incredible wins. Think as well about the things and people that have helped you along the way.

Over the next few pages, try to complete the exercises as best you can. These will help you see just how much you've achieved when you come back to them.

"Anxiety is a very individual journey that's probably had many ups and downs"

EXPRESS YOURSELF

Studies show that journaling can help you reduce symptoms of anxiety, as writing it all down helps you to process your emotions.

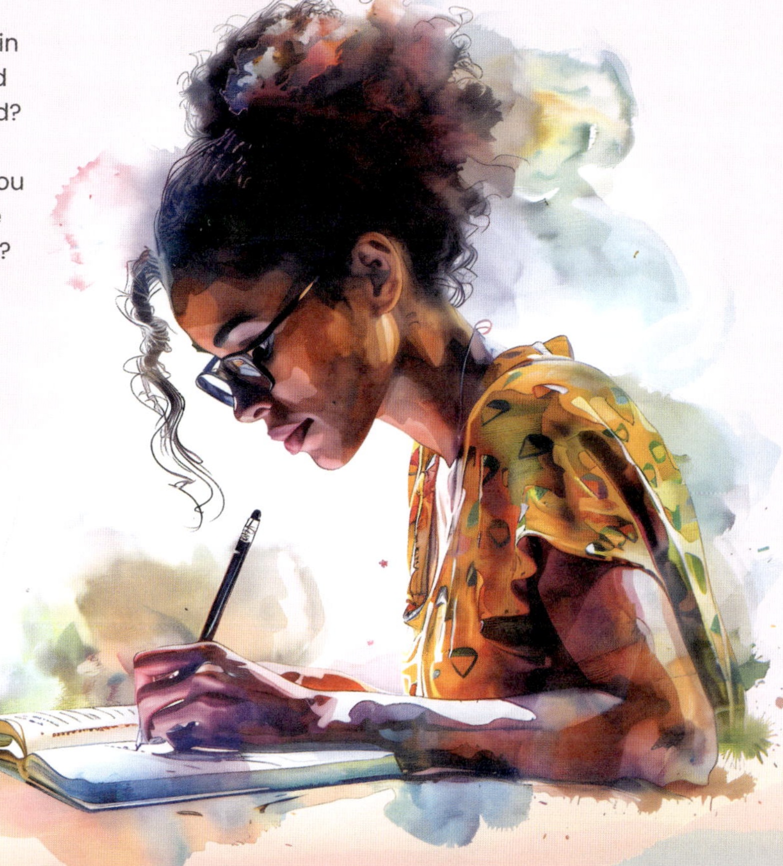

MY ANXIETIES

MY SYMPTOMS

PATTERNS IN YOUR ANXIETY

Think about how you deal with anxiety, and you might start to see some patterns arise. This could be triggers that make your anxiety worse, or maybe you find your anxiety is heightened on certain days of the week, times of the month, or seasons of the year. Maybe you notice a completely different pattern. Use this page to make a note of these patterns, as they can help you to plan for managing your anxiety.

TRIGGER PATTERNS

- ◇
- ◇
- ◇
- ◇
- ◇

TIME PERIOD PATTERNS

- ◇
- ◇
- ◇
- ◇
- ◇

OTHER PATTERNS

- ◇
- ◇
- ◇
- ◇
- ◇

HOW DO YOU DEAL WITH ANXIETY?

SITUATION

How did I react?

Outcome

SITUATION

How did I react?

Outcome

SITUATION

How did I react?

Outcome

CHALLENGES AND LESSONS

What challenges have you faced this year? When you have anxiety, things that challenge you might seem small to someone else, but it's how much they affect you that matters. Think about some of the obstacles and difficulties you've faced and what you did, then come back to this section at the end of the book and consider any lessons you've learned to take into the future.

CHALLENGE

What I did

Lessons learned

CHALLENGE

What I did

Lessons learned

CHALLENGE

What I did

Lessons learned

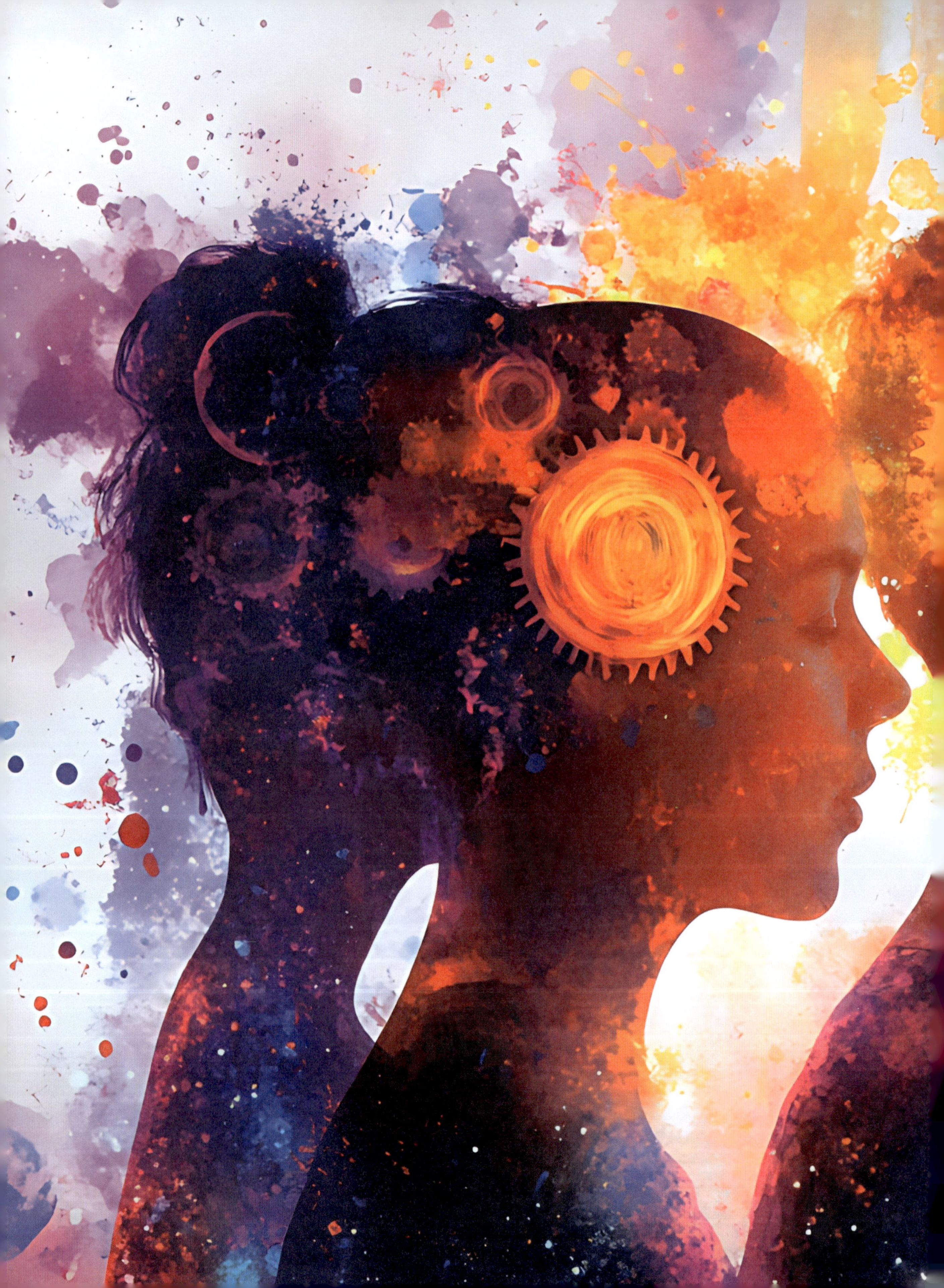

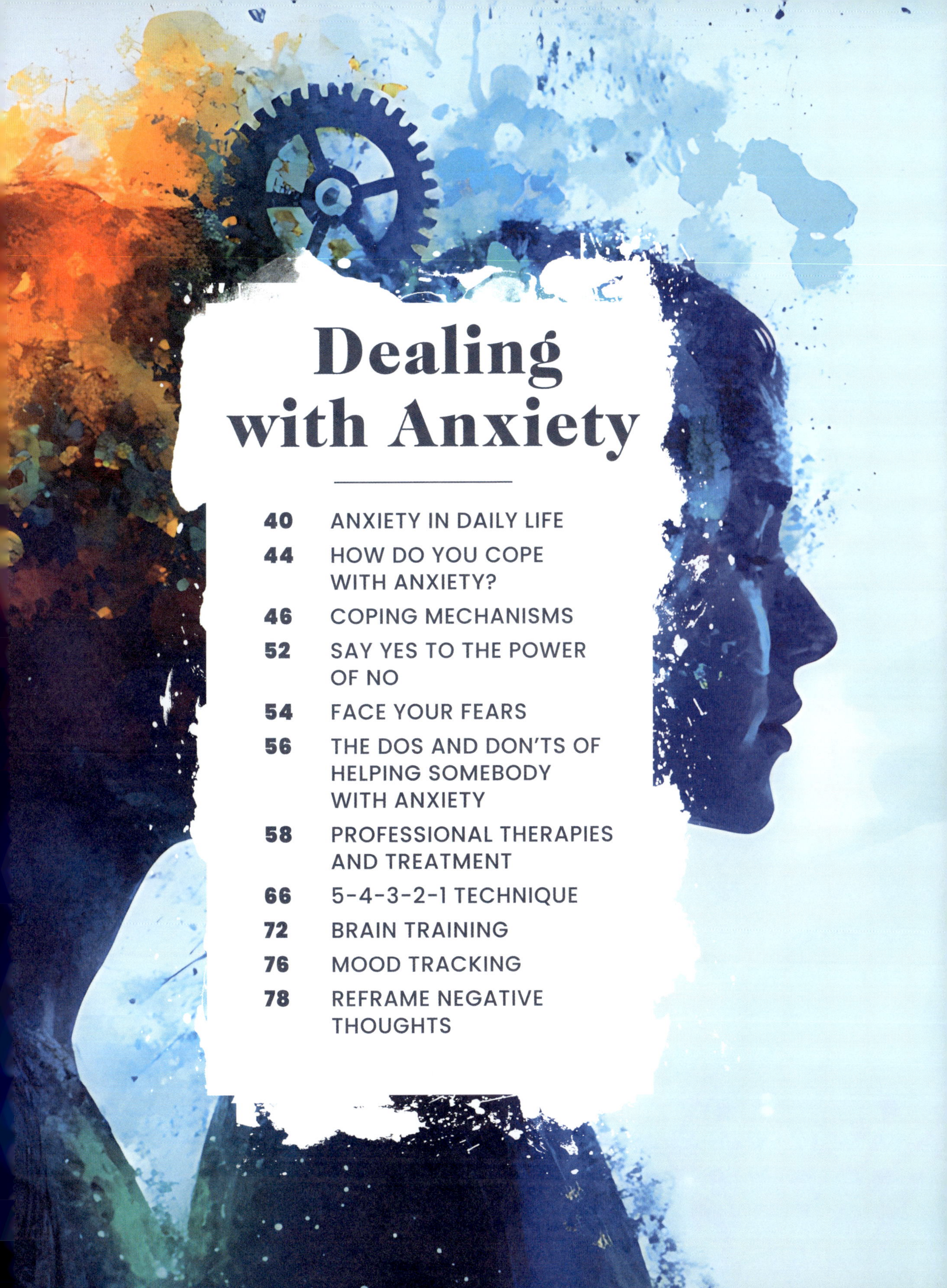

Dealing with Anxiety

Anxiety in Daily Life

ANXIETY CAN REAR ITS UGLY HEAD IN ALL MANNER OF SITUATIONS; HERE'S HOW TO DEAL WITH IT IN SOME OF THE MORE COMMON ONES.

Anxiety is the body's alarm, activated by perceived threats. Sometimes we learn or become attuned to these triggers—things or places that could set us off—and create coping strategies to deal with them, thus deactivating the alarm. However, there can be times when the mental and physical symptoms of anxiety take us by surprise, and are often more challenging to control.

In both circumstances it's vital to remember that anxiety can be tamed. Whether it's through self-care, mindfulness, support groups, therapy, or where appropriate, medication, there are plenty of things we can do to control our anxiety.

Within this feature, we explore six common situations that are most likely to create anxious behavior, and offer specific coping strategies for each. What's more, because the mind is such a powerful tool, you might find these techniques can be transferred to a wider range of situations and environments, helping you to take control any time, any place, whether it's preemptively or when anxiety strikes most unexpectedly.

SOCIAL SITUATIONS

Parties, get-togethers, or even hobbies or activities you may want to try naturally increase stress levels, because apprehension of the unfamiliar is part of the survival instinct left over from our cave-dwelling days. Remind yourself that only you can control whether you have a good time, and so reframe any negative thoughts before you even leave the house; for example, "I'm too shy" becomes "I'm going to be braver today," or "I'm too nervous to go" changes to "I feel excited." In the moment, push yourself to stand more centrally than you have in the past, or be more curious about other people than you were before; even marginal improvements go a long way to easing tension. Avoid negative coping strategies like drinking too much alcohol to "get through it" and don't be tempted to sideline yourself; use the stress like an athlete uses adrenaline to push for personal growth and improvement.

SOCIAL MEDIA

If social media is stressing you out, ask yourself—do you need it? If it's taking more than it's giving, delete your accounts and live a less burdened lifestyle. If that's not possible, perhaps try diminishing the impact it has by turning off notifications, "hiding" the app deep in a folder, or only allow yourself certain amounts of time to use them, such as five minutes per hour, or half an hour at a time where you have no more responsibilities: the commute home on public transportation or when your children are in bed. Set a timer, because it's all too easy to get sucked in, and if you start experiencing anxiety or get upset, remind yourself that people only ever

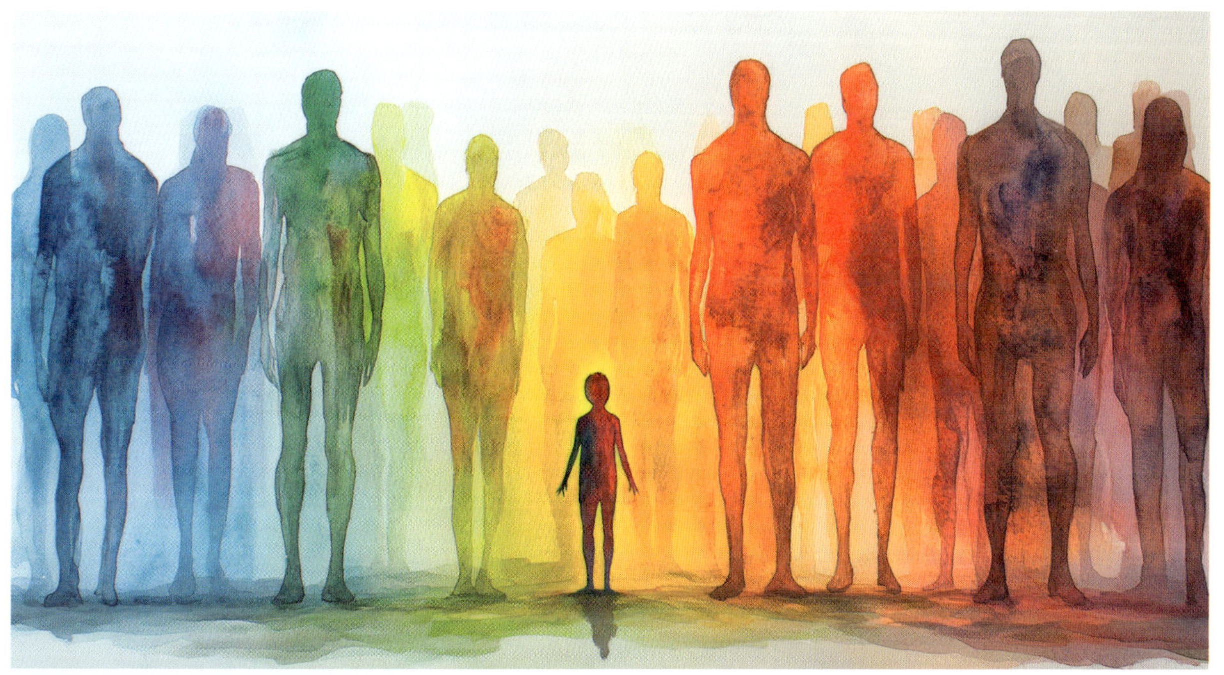

use these apps to boost, provoke, or highlight their experiences. Very little of what you see on social media actually comes from a positive place.

IN THE HOME

From the color of a wall to constant clutter, distracting noises to flickering lights, even seemingly innocuous household objects like a clock—there are many things in the home that can trigger anxiety. The way to deal with this is to change what's within your control. If something is triggering you—change it. Paint over that bright red wall with a more soothing shade, or if you rent, put up removable wallpaper! Chuck out those scales, and change that light fitting. Control your surroundings and you'll help to control your anxiety. If it's your environment that's setting you off, change that as well. Introduce houseplants—which are proven to relax and positively stimulate—declutter, add soft furnishings, or use an air diffuser with a scent that centers you. Simply put, create calm from what was previously chaos.

AT WORK

The workplace (or school) can create a lot of anxiety, whether it's feeling out of your comfort zone, wielding little control or input into how a role is performed, being in a toxic environment

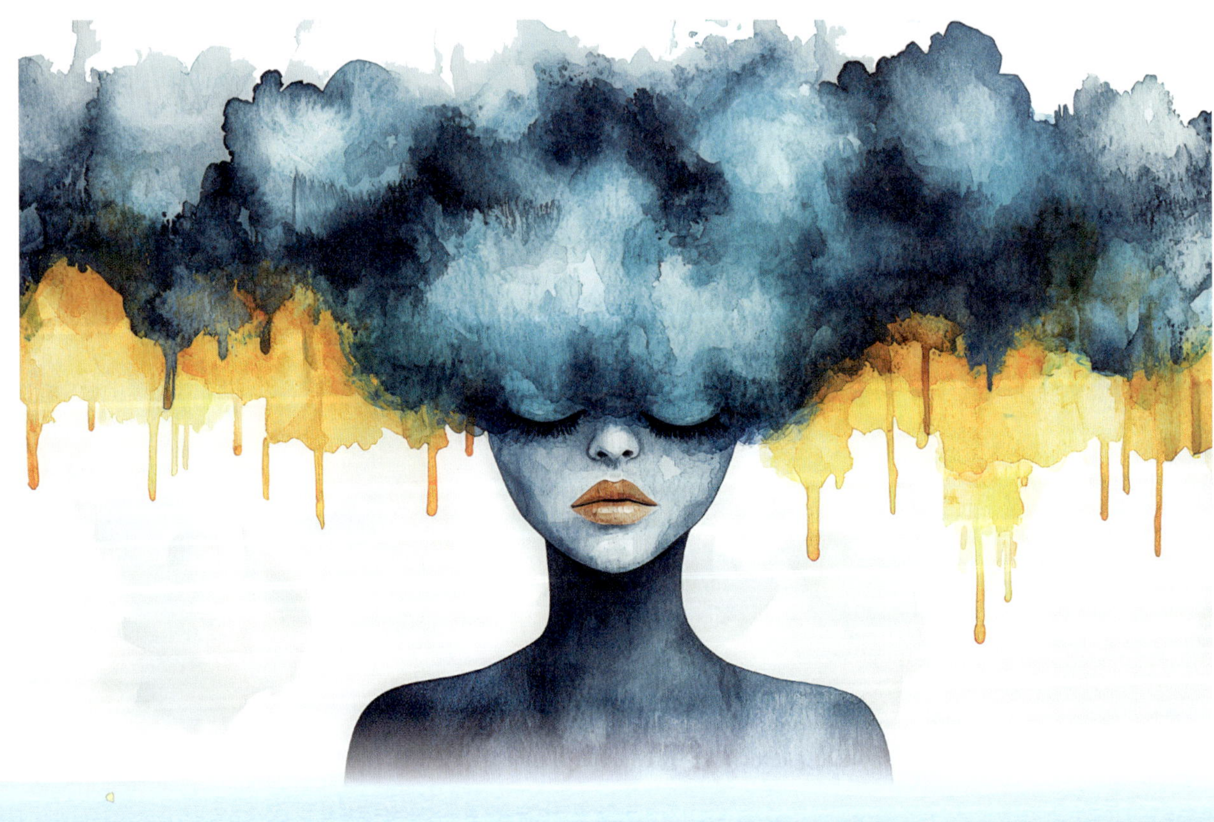

"Whether it's a crowded train or peak shopping time at the local supermarket, there are coping mechanisms you can employ to recenter"

where conflict is an everyday occurrence, a lack of recognition of your hard work, or a change that has left you unsettled. Whatever the stressor, you can calm your anxiety by finding ways to deal with the pressure and improve your ability to cope. First, accept that you can only control what you do and how you react. If you have a problem with someone at work, talk to them, and if nothing changes, contact your human resources department. If you're feeling overwhelmed, take back control by starting each day with a routine of prioritizing and planning out your working hours. When the work day ends, mentally train yourself to leave it all behind. If you think of something outside of work, make a quick note for the next day, and mentally move on.

BUSY AND/OR CROWDED PLACES

Busy places can threaten our sense of control, which increases stress levels. But whether it's a crowded train or peak shopping time at the local supermarket, there are coping mechanisms you can employ to recenter. If you feel overwhelmed, take back control; close your eyes and focus on the ground beneath your feet, or distract yourself by mentally talking through what you can see, rather than focusing on how it makes you feel. Look to calm any loud or distracting stimuli; for example, animated voices on a train—it's in your power to pop on headphones and enjoy music that helps you relax. Likewise, minimize distracting or unpleasant smells by adding a drop of your favorite essential oil onto the end of your sleeve or a hankie, then smell it. Not only will the scent lower

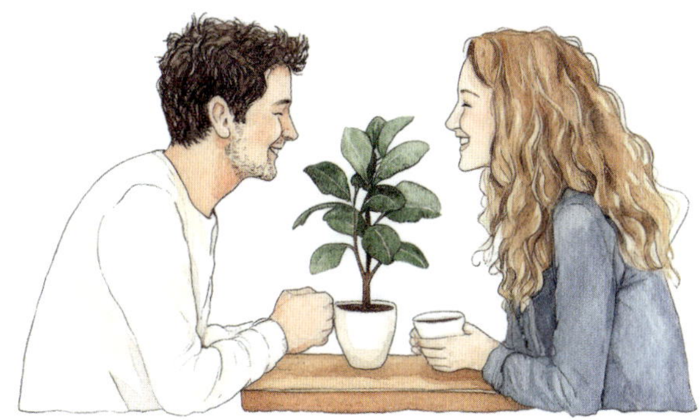

your stress levels, but it will also help to regulate your breathing and lower your heart rate.

DATING

Fear of the unknown plus fear of rejection can stir anxious feelings before, during, and after a date, for some even manifesting physically (such as excessive sweating, nausea, or an accelerated heartbeat). Cope with these feelings by communicating openly and honestly with your date. If you feel you need to be the one that makes the plans, then express that. If you feel more comfortable with people you know, suggest a double or group date. If things start to overwhelm you, explain what's happening or take a few moments by excusing yourself to go outside to practice some mindfulness techniques, slowing your breathing and lowering a racing heart.

How Do You Cope with Anxiety?

DETERMINE WHAT TYPE OF COPING MECHANISMS YOU'RE CURRENTLY USING WHEN ANXIOUS.

There are different ways of coping when faced with anxiety; some will try to avoid situations that make them feel anxious, while others will seek to control a situation through careful planning. Some will look for comfort and support from friends and family, while others will take a more proactive approach. There are no wrong answers here; be honest about what you do when faced with an anxious situation, as this will help identify your current coping style. This helps you learn what's effective for you, as well as what's detrimental to your well-being.

A BIT OF EVERYTHING

If you've checked a mix of answers, it might be that you use different strategies in different situations. Think about which ones work the best for you and what areas/situations you need to improve upon.

QUIZ

When I'm feeling the effects of anxiety, I usually:

A Bury my head in the sand—ignoring it or going to bed to sleep it off

B Research all the symptoms to reassure myself that everything is under control

C Talk to a trusted friend or family member to make sure I'm okay

D Take a moment to acknowledge the feeling and use calming techniques, such as breathing exercises

When a big social event is coming up, I tend to:

A Not think about it and distract myself on my phone or by watching TV

B Make lists to ensure I've thought of everything I need to do to prepare

C Phone or text a friend to talk through the event and what I should be doing

D Reflect on what's making me feel anxious about the event, and take a pause to work through it

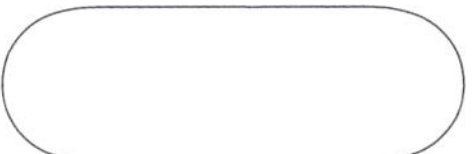

When I'm anxious, I try to make myself feel better by:

A Avoiding whatever is making me anxious

B Planning, researching, or scheduling my day so I feel more in control

C Asking someone else to reassure me that everything is okay

D Working through the triggers and causes to understand why I'm feeling anxious

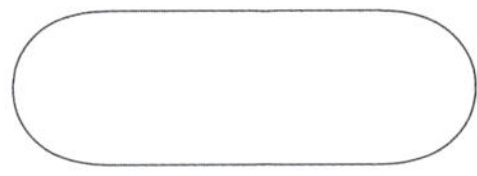

When I'm feeling overwhelmed, I tend to:

A Cancel plans and withdraw into myself in a safe space

B Go over my plans or do more research to make sure that I haven't missed anything

C Talk to a few different people to get some advice and some reassurance

D Do a calming activity or some mindful movement

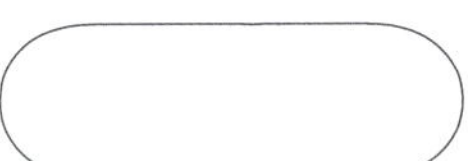

MOSTLY As

Avoid—you tend to back away from anxiety triggers through denial or avoidance. While this can initially help, your anxiety can pile up—you need to learn how to face your triggers and tolerate the discomfort.

MOSTLY Bs

Control—you like to be in control, using planning and lists to manage anxiety; however this can mean that you get more anxious when things don't go to plan. You need to embrace being more flexible.

MOSTLY Cs

Validate—you rely on external validation and comfort from your friends and family to ease your anxiety. While it's great you have a good support system, you need to trust your own judgment as well.

MOSTLY Ds

Process—you have healthy, balanced coping strategies to manage your anxiety. You're on the right path, but don't forget to make time to rest and relax.

CONCLUSION

By understanding how you react to anxiety, you can find coping strategies.

Coping Mechanisms

THERE ARE MANY TECHNIQUES YOU CAN USE TO COPE WITH ANXIETY; WE EXPLORE SOME OF THEM HERE.

Having anxiety can feel overwhelming at times, and it can be hard to think straight or calm down when you're in the midst of it. In times like these, it helps to have a set of strategies to ground you and bring you back to the present moment, giving you a chance to reset, relax, and regain control. Here we explore five different coping mechanisms for you to try.

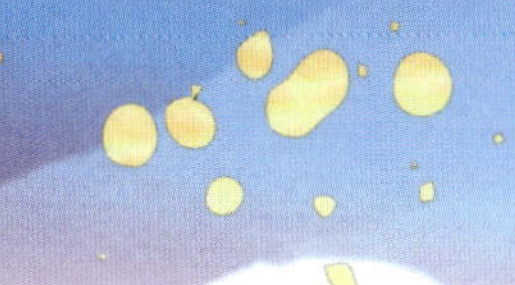

BREATHING TECHNIQUES

A really simple way to manage your anxiety is to harness breathing exercises. You might find it useful to do a breathing exercise every day as part of your daily routine, which can help to stop anxiety from building up. Alternatively, you can learn breathing exercises that will help you in the moment when you're feeling particularly anxious. Some people find it beneficial to do a breathing exercise before bed, as it can help to calm the mind for sleep. Whenever you choose to do them, there are many different breathing exercises available, but they all essentially do the same thing, which is to help you focus mindfully on your breath as you inhale and exhale. Doing this gives you a chance to pause, calm down, and slow your breathing. If you've never tried a breathing exercise before, start simple. Make sure you're sitting or lying somewhere comfortably where you won't be disturbed. Breathe deeply in through your nose and out through your mouth. If you find your breathing is rapid, try to count to five both as you inhale and as you exhale. Continue doing this for a few minutes until you feel more regulated. Once you've got the hang of this, you can try other breathing exercises and patterns. For example, box breathing involves inhaling for four counts, holding the breath for four counts, exhaling for four counts, and then holding again for another four counts. Some people like to visualize the sides of a box when they're doing this, hence the name. Another common pattern is 4-7-8, which means inhaling through your nose for four seconds, holding your breath for seven seconds, before exhaling through your mouth for eight seconds. Try a few different patterns to find the one that works for you.

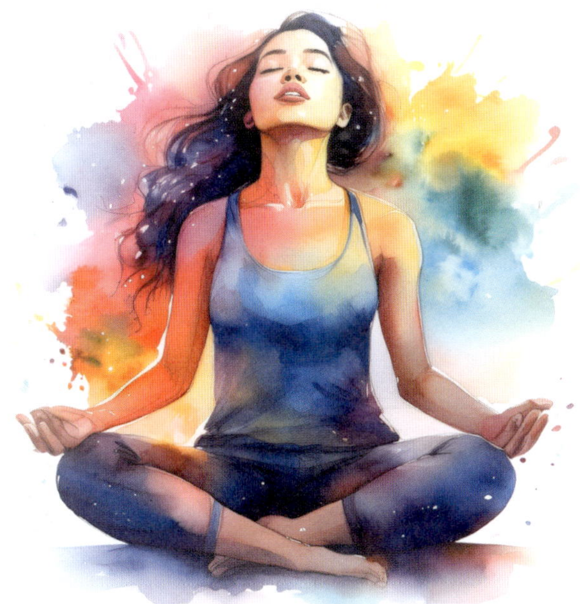

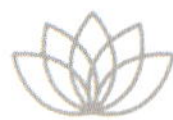

GROUNDING EXERCISES

When you're experiencing a state of anxiety, it isn't unusual to feel a bit untethered from the world around you, which can heighten your worry and panic. This is where "grounding" comes in. Grounding means to anchor or tether yourself to the present moment, which is an excellent way of shifting your focus away from whatever is worrying you or flooding your thoughts, and enabling you to feel calmer and more in control. One simple grounding technique that's commonly used by people who are anxious or feeling panicked is the 5-4-3-2-1 method. This involves stretching your senses out to the world around you and looking for five things you can see, four things you can touch, three things you can hear, two things you can smell, and one thing you can taste. In truth, the numbers don't really matter that much; it's the principle of focusing on the information your senses are receiving. Therefore, if you'd rather just find one thing for each sense, or five things for each sense, that's absolutely fine. If you have a very busy brain, another technique is to describe your surroundings. Look around you and think about everything that you can see, right down to the smallest detail. For example, rather than just thinking "I see a cup," you would think "I see a red cup with a floral pattern and a chink on the left side." It's the level of detail that helps to shift your focus away from the anxious and negative thoughts toward your present environment. Other people, however, may prefer to use more physical grounding techniques, for example stomping your feet on the ground or making fists with your hands and then releasing them.

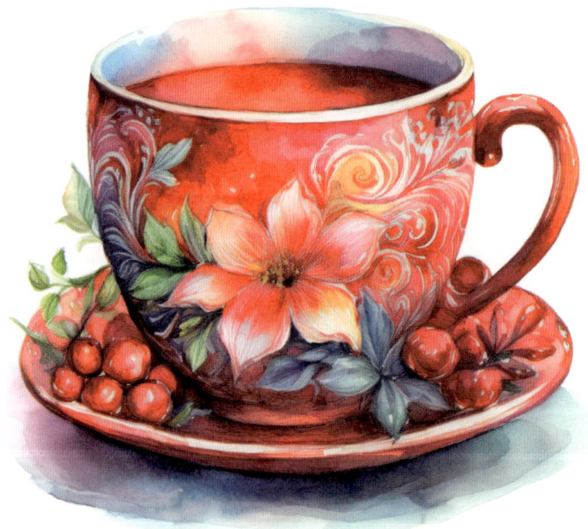

PROGRESSIVE MUSCLE RELAXATION (PMR)

PMR is an excellent technique for relaxation, which can help to ease the physical symptoms of anxiety. The process also helps to focus your brain, which can stop negative thoughts from spiraling and connect you with the present moment. It also encourages you to become more aware of your body and where you hold tension, so is an excellent exercise for tackling multiple problem areas. The idea is that you actively tense different parts of your body, hold that tension for a few seconds, and then release it. You then do the same again in a different area of the body. Most people prefer to do this in a logical order, for example by starting with the head and moving down to the toes, or vice versa. Having a sequence that you copy every time you do PMR can help to create a pattern that your body adapts to, meaning it can calm your anxiety more quickly as you know what to expect. There are many known benefits of PMR, including reduced stress and anxiety, better sleep, and even helping with cognitive function. The most important elements of performing PMR are comfort and consistency. Make sure you can lie somewhere comfortably, using cushions if you need to secure your body in an optimum position. Try to create a habit of performing PMR regularly to really benefit from it. If you have any areas of your body where you have an injury or pain for whatever reason, you may find you can't tense that area and it's better to skip it—PMR should cause no pain.

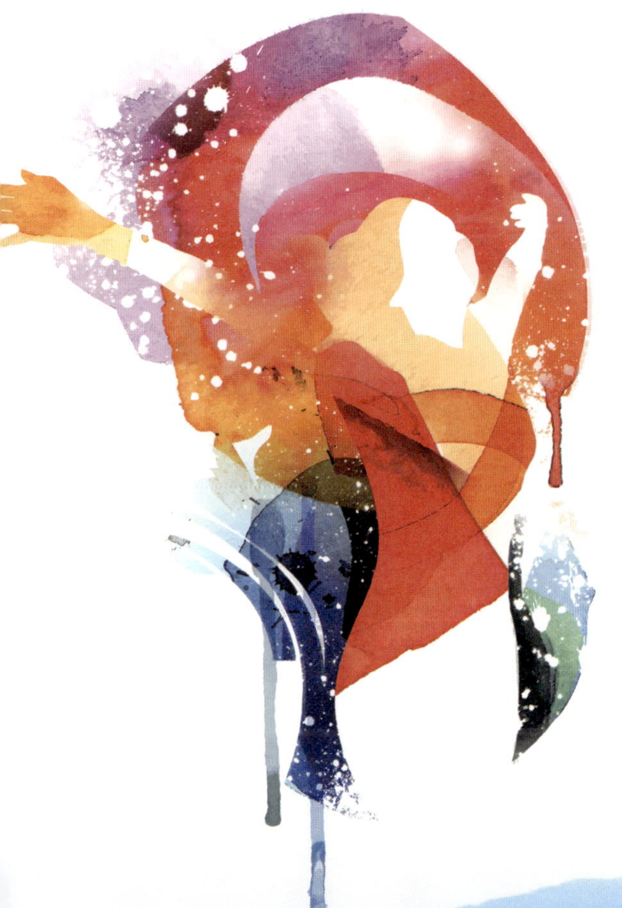

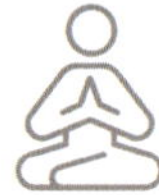

MINDFULNESS AND MEDITATION

Both mindfulness and meditation can be powerful strategies to keep in your mental toolbox. Mindfulness is a state of mind in which you are present, connected with the world around you, and aware of your thoughts and feelings. You can apply mindfulness to pretty much all of your everyday activities. For example, when you go for a walk, you can train yourself to be mindful about your environment—focusing on what you can see and hear. Additionally, when you're eating a meal you can be mindful about the taste, flavor, and texture of the food. Meditation, on the other hand, is a specific practice or activity, usually structured or guided, to help you achieve a state of mindfulness and attention. It can be useful to bring elements of both into your daily life to help manage your anxiety. For instance, you may wish to add a formal meditative practice into your routine, whether that's first thing in the morning as a way of setting your intentions for the day, or last thing at night to calm your mind for sleep. At the same time, you may wish to also introduce mindfulness into your everyday life to help you maintain that quiet focus and engagement. If you've never meditated before it can take a little practice, as it involves quietening your mind, and letting thoughts drift in and out, but not feeling caught up in them. A simple meditative technique is called the "body scan," where you mentally scan up and down your body, focusing on different parts and tuning in to how they feel. Some people prefer to opt for guided meditation, which could be in person, with a teacher, or using an app that talks you through an exercise from start to finish.

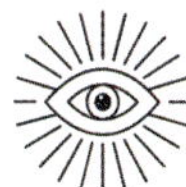

VISUALIZATION

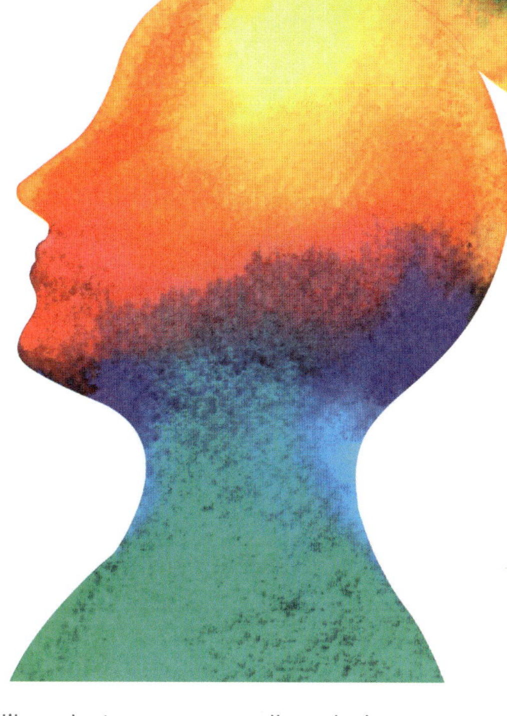

If you're a very visual and creative person, visualization is another technique that you can try to help manage your anxiety. This means creating and crafting mental imagery that helps you to feel more relaxed and calmer. By creating a detailed visualization, it helps to move your brain away from anxious and negative thoughts. It can temporarily distract you from what you're worrying about, giving you a chance to calm down, and can reduce stress and heightened emotions. A calming visualization can also trigger responses in the brain that help you to feel more relaxed, such as slower, deeper breathing and a lower heart rate. Visualization can be based around creating a place in your mind where you feel safe. This could be a real place that makes you feel happy and secure, and you can draw on your real-life experience to bring this visual to life in great detail. Some people may create a fictional place using elements of what they find calming, such as a forest, a beach, or a rolling country landscape. When building your visualization, bring in information about what you can see, what it feels like, what you can smell, and what you can hear. Some people find it hard to build detailed visuals like this, but that doesn't mean you can't use visualization. You may find it easier to visualize a golden thread connecting you to the ground to help anchor you in the present. Or maybe you can visualize breathing in a calming light and breathing out the dark shadows of anxiety. You can also get guided imagery exercises that encourage you to create certain scenes or environments, and these can be good for getting to grips with the technique.

BUILD YOUR REGIME

Are you drawn to any of these techniques more than others? Which ones do you feel are the most effective? You may find that a combination of strategies works best in different situations.

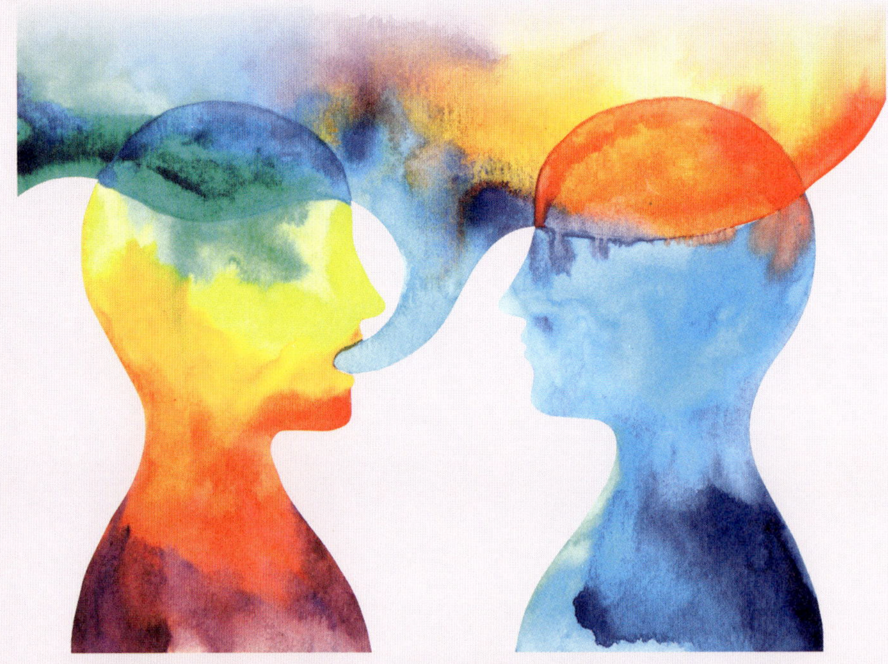

SAY YES TO THE POWER OF NO!

Agreeing to everything may keep others happy, but often at a personal cost. Here's why setting boundaries and sometimes saying no means saying yes to self-worth.

Growing up, we are generally taught that saying no all the time is considered impolite. And while young children have no problem using the word freely, sometimes as adults we need reminding of our right to it.

It's one thing to want to help others, but people who feel as though they simply can't say no suffer from an uncontrollable need for approval, and they may have deep-seated fears of anger and confrontation. As the late, acclaimed psychologist Dr. Harriet Braiker points out in *The Disease to Please: Curing the People-Pleasing Syndrome*: "For many, the difficulty may start innocently enough with genuine and generous attempts to make others happy. But this seemingly harmless passion to always be 'nice,' to put others first and to compulsively please them even at the expense of your own health and happiness rapidly spirals into a serious psychological syndrome with far-reaching physical and emotional consequences."

It's obvious that continually adding to a heavy workload because you can't say no to anything risks causing physical exhaustion. But we are less likely to consider how emotionally unhealthy it is too. Always shelving our own needs and desires to meet someone else's sends out the message that we don't deserve any—both to ourselves, as well as others, who may take advantage of this. Of course, there are numerous situations where agreeing to things we don't want to do is inevitable.

If your teenager calls to say they are stranded, safety concerns will override the fact that being woken at 3:00 a.m. to drive into town wasn't on our agenda. For somebody struggling financially, turning down paid overtime may not feel like an option, however much they have on their plate. But if there's the expectation you'll drop your own plans to provide a regular unpaid taxi service, or to work late every time a report is dropped on your desk at 5:00 p.m., learning how to say no is an essential skill for you to master.

For those suffering from the "please disease," this may take some groundwork. First, you need to assess why you continually agree to things you don't want to do. What does no represent? Is it rejection from social circles? A fear of being disliked, or not doing your job properly? Or a concern for being seen as a "bad" parent or partner? Did you grow up seeing it as essential to toe the line to avoid difficult situations? Remind yourself that self-care is not the same as being selfish, and it isn't your job to take on everyone else's problems. If low self-esteem is the issue, work on this with a counselor. Then follow our tips for regaining the right to say no:

Start small. Like any habit, saying yes to everything can be hard to break. Some people will feel easier to say no to than others, just as some things will—start with these and build up.

–

Give yourself time. If your default response is to immediately agree, say that you need to check arrangements. Just don't let this turn into procrastination and guilt.

–

Focus on the positives of a negative and your desired outcome. Saying no to something that isn't a fit for you means being able to say yes to something that is.

–

Be prepared for some people to be taken aback or try to persuade you. Stay polite but firm.

Avoid rambling explanations. "That sounds lovely but I have plans on Friday" is enough. As etiquette expert and author Judith Martin once acknowledged: "Part of the skill of saying no is to shut up afterwards and not babble on, offering material for an argument."

Give an alternative suggestion if there's a compromise that works for you, as long as you don't end up agreeing to something else that doesn't. It's pointless saying no to manning a stand at a fête, only to get lumbered with making cupcakes when you don't have time for either.

Finally, if you regularly struggle with how to answer a request or demand, heed this simple line of advice from Brazilian novelist Paulo Coelho: "If you must say yes, say it with an open heart. If you must say no, say it without fear."

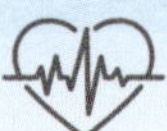

FACE YOUR FEARS!

Does a fear of flying stop you from booking a vacation? Do you hate driving so therefore haven't seen friends for ages? You're not alone. A report by John Hopkins Medicine found that 19 million people in the United States have a phobia, with many of us avoiding certain places because of it. "Phobias are a type of fear, but are irrational or extreme, where the potential danger of a certain situation or object is exaggerated," says Dr. Mark Winwood, director of psychological services for AXA PPP Healthcare. "The thought can be paralyzing."

WHAT MAKES US SUSCEPTIBLE?

So why do some of us get affected by such anxieties? "We're actually only born with two fears—the fear of falling and loud noises," says Dr. Winwood. "All others are learned." Known as a "learned response," phobias have been caused by a shocking or traumatic event, which then develops into an aversion to anything associated with the memory.

"For some people, the origins of why we are phobic is less clear," says psychotherapist Toby Ingham. "We don't remember the particular experience, all we know is that we may have been left with the residual sense of fear."

TIME TO CHANGE

However it started, it's important to remember that fear is a natural response to a threat to survival—it's there to protect us. "If we can think about our fears differently, we can see them as a positive, motivating force," says Dr. Winwood. "The first step is identifying what our fears are and the function of them. The more we can understand them, we can stop them from limiting us. We can then stop our fears disabling us, and feel empowered." Here's how:

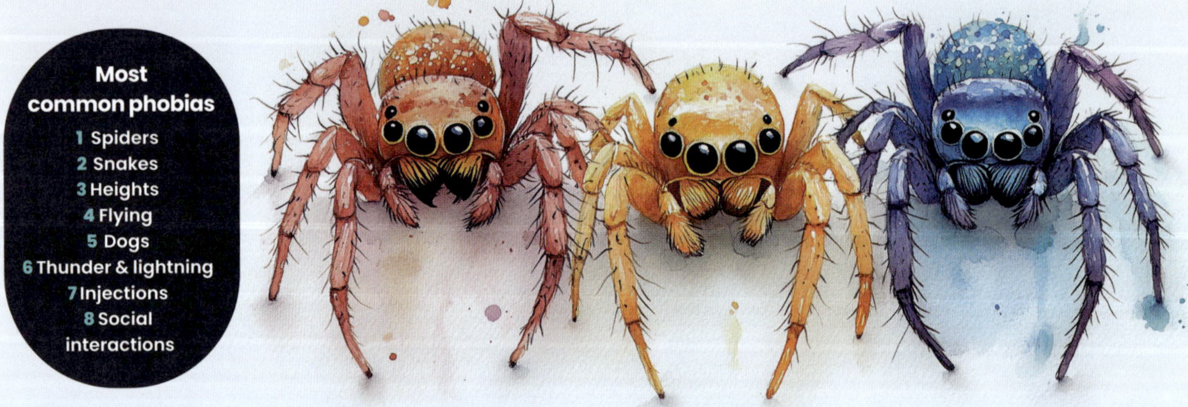

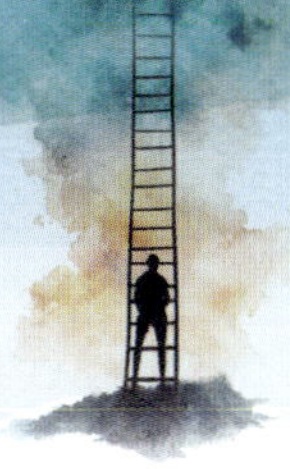

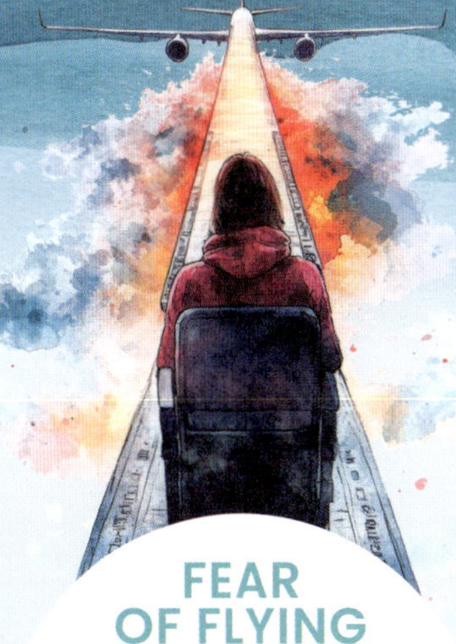

FEAR OF HEIGHTS

"Acrophobia is rooted in a fear that we'll lose control," says Dr. Winwood. "It's natural to feel nervous from an unnatural height—genetically speaking, keeping away from dangerous drops was an evolutionary necessity."

Cure it: **"Slowly exposing yourself to new heights, such as looking over a stairwell, is a strong starting point," explains Dr. Winwood. "When you're feeling braver, you could try an experience day involving a zip line or indoor skydiving. Cognitive behavioral therapy (CBT) could help train your brain into thinking of heights as a perceived threat that you're in control of."**

FEAR OF DRIVING

Driving anxiety can start gradually, after an accident or near miss, or can be linked to a fear in your own ability to take control. If you're also menopausal, fluctuating hormones could be to blame. "If you were a rather anxious driver before, the physical and cognitive symptoms of the menopause could make driving feel even more scary," says psychologist Dr. Meg Arroll.

Cure it: **Start with small trips or try difficult journeys with a friend first. "It's important to discover what it is about driving that actually creates the fear," says Lorna Cordwell from Chrysalis Courses UK. "When driving is criticized by others, it destroys confidence. This is an issue that can be explored in therapy."**

FEAR OF FLYING

Also known as aerophobia, it affects more than 25 million people in the United States, while studies show 7 to 15 percent of American adults suffer from a specific phobia in their lifetime. "This stems from thinking about external factors that are beyond your control, such as turbulence, bad weather, or an engineering fault," says Dr. Winwood. "People with aerophobia are acutely aware that if the plane encounters trouble they are helpless."

Cure it: **"Acknowledge it—seeking out alternative methods of travel only reinforces the phobia," says Dr. Winwood. "Anxiety thrives off 'what if?' catastrophic thoughts, so we can help overcome this by brushing up on the facts. Research how a plane flies and the causes of turbulence, so you know what to expect. That can help give you a feeling of greater control over the risk. Online flight simulators can also be helpful and many airlines offer special courses. Alternatively, therapists can also suggest breathing techniques to help you stay calm." Try the Headspace app for easy breathing exercises that can be used offline.**

FEAR OF SPIDERS

"Arachnophobia may link to our earliest experience of spotting signs of danger, of surprise attack, of infection and disease," says Toby Ingham. "It's partly to do with the sense that there is suddenly something there that wasn't invited."

Cure it: **"For some people it's very hard to relax when you know a spider is in the room, particularly if it suddenly disappears," says Ingham. "But gradually exposing yourself to spiders can take the shock value away. Take deep breaths, concentrate on calming yourself, and remember the spider is very small compared to you. There are apps, for example, Arachnophobia Free (iOS), which create a virtual way of learning to relax when it comes to spiders."**

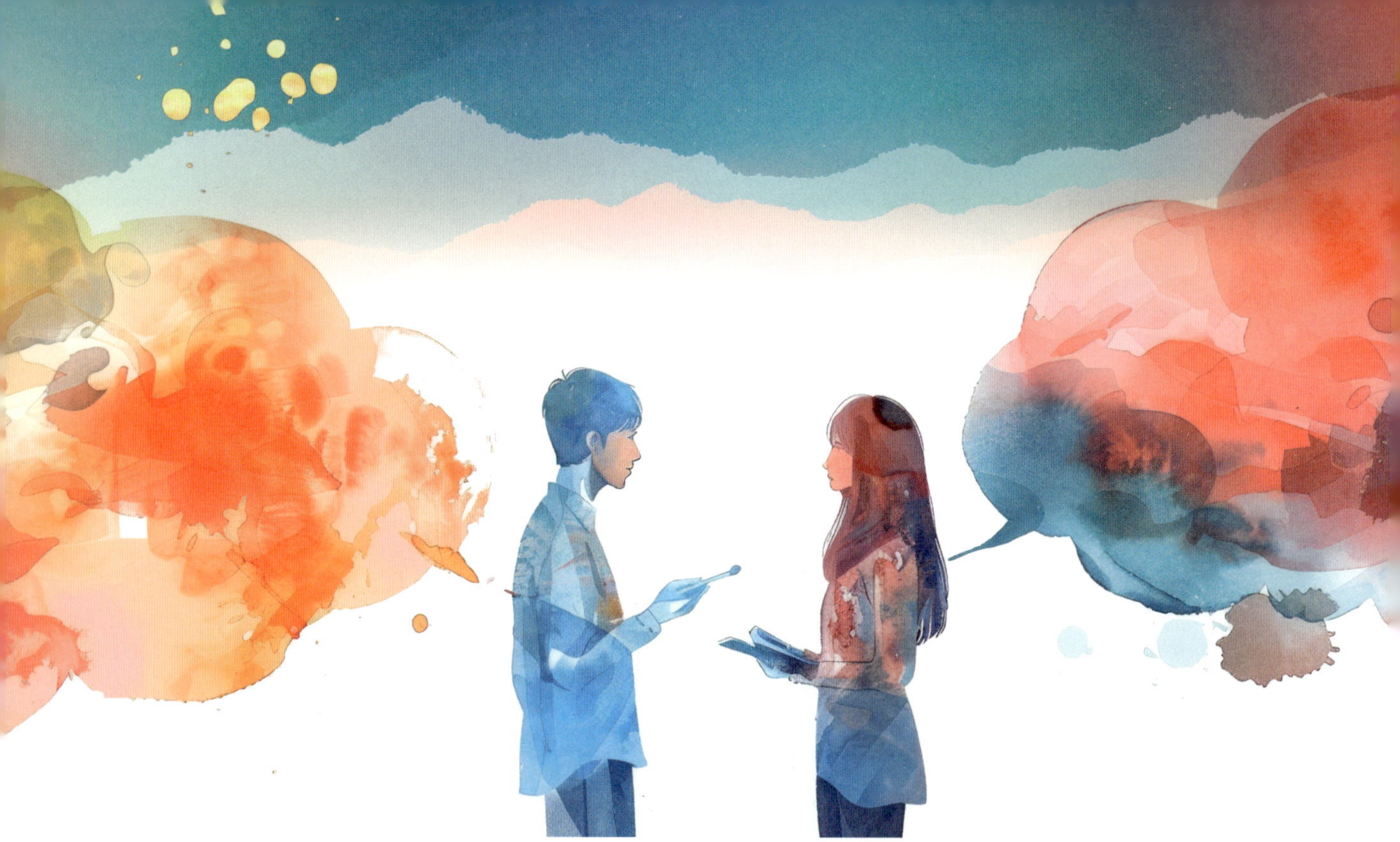

THE DOS AND DON'TS OF HELPING SOMEBODY WITH ANXIETY

If somebody close to you is suffering from anxiety, offer the best support possible with these top tips.

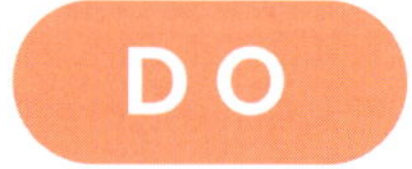

Take the pressure off
If a friend or colleague is struggling with tasks at home or at work, and you are able to help alleviate their stress by taking on some of their workload, this support may help reduce their anxiety.

Validate their feelings
Acknowledging and accepting how an anxious person is feeling can make them feel seen and understood. Research also suggests validation helps people better regulate their emotions.

Offer your support
Letting somebody with anxiety know you are there for them can come as a welcome relief. Just be sure to listen to how exactly they wish to be supported.

Be available
Let your loved one know that they can talk to you at any time without fear of judgment. Providing reassurance that your overall perception of them will not change is sure to help too.

Look after yourself
Helping somebody you care about with anxiety can be tough, so it's important to prioritize your own self-care. By keeping yourself well, you're in a much better position to offer support.

Educate yourself
Learning about the different types of anxiety and how different symptoms manifest can help you understand what the person you care about is going through.

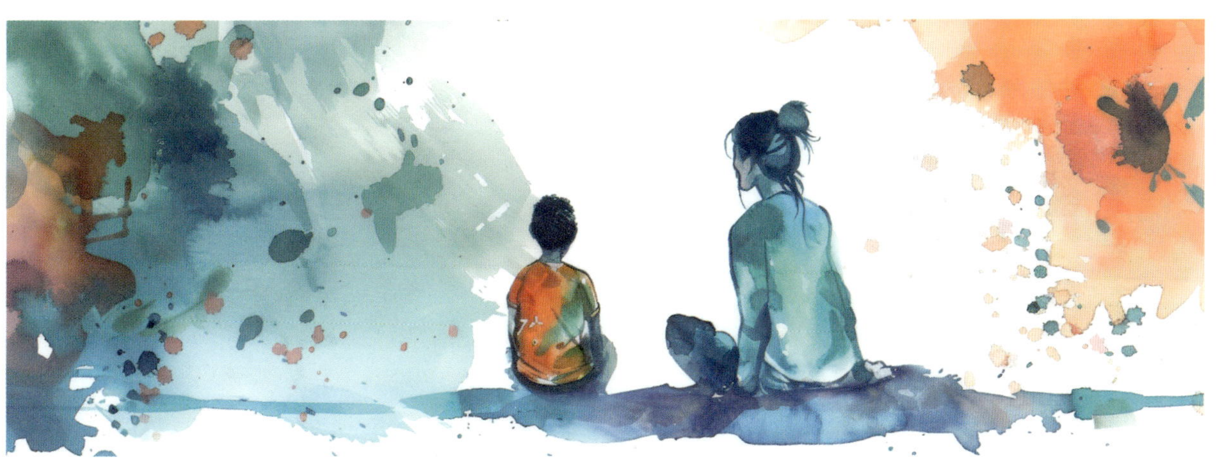

DON'T

Expect immediate change
Recovering from an anxiety disorder is often a long process. Remember to be patient as your loved one learns the strategies and techniques they need to heal.

Do it alone
You won't always be able to help a friend or family member with anxiety. In some cases, encouraging them to access professional support and therapy is crucial for their recovery.

Get frustrated
People suffering from high levels of anxiety often struggle to engage with their work, social activities, hobbies, and more. Try not to take their avoidance personally.

Enable their anxiety
Make sure you're not helping the person avoid certain anxiety-inducing situations. Although this avoidance might seem helpful in the short term, it will end up having a negative impact in the long run.

Tell them to calm down
The phrase "calm down'" implies that somebody is simply not choosing to control their anxiety. As a result, the instruction can cause feelings of shame, loneliness, and powerlessness—not helpful.

Professional Therapies & Treatment

WHETHER TO EASE RECURRING SYMPTOMS OR PINPOINT MAJOR UNDERLYING ISSUES, THESE METHODS CAN TARGET AND CONTROL ANXIETY DISORDERS.

Seeking professional help for anxiety might seem like the hardest leap to take. While you're battling to regain control of your body and its consuming mental and physical feelings of anxiety, surrendering more control to a professional can be daunting.

However, approaching a mental health expert and allowing them to make the best decision for your anxiety disorder can ensure that you are able to take back greater control of your life in the long term.

There are many therapies and treatments that are designed to reduce the symptoms of anxiety. The three main types are medication, psychotherapy, and daily management. If anxiety is a regular part of your life, a combination of these methods can be used together to transform your quality of life.

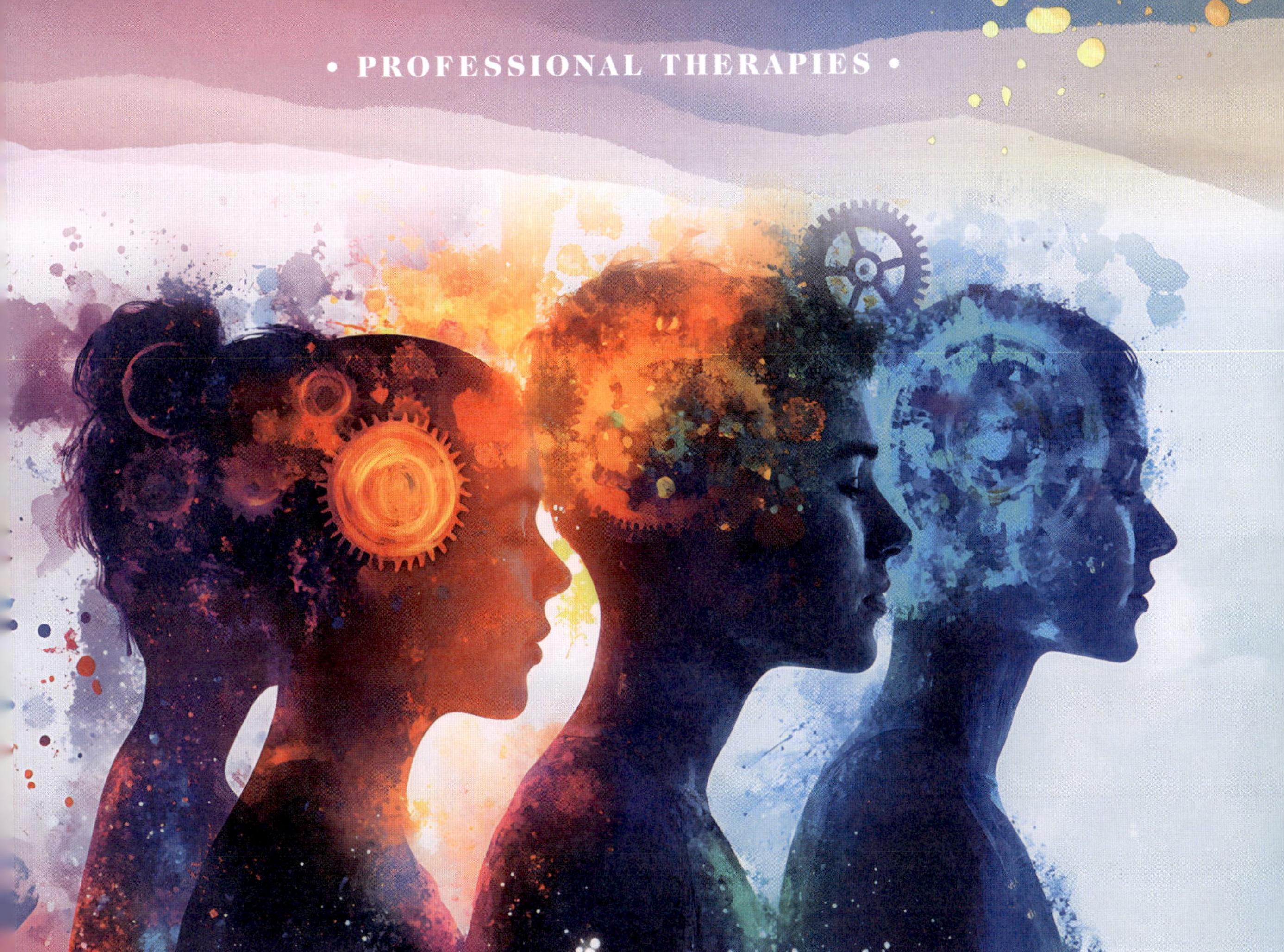

Knowing the personal triggers for your anxiety attacks means that you can try to manage your exposure to them. However, this pressure alone can sometimes impact your mental health further. With the help of professionals, it's possible to take the driving seat in your life—to delve into the root causes of your anxiety and establish longer-lasting ways to put anxiety in the back seat.

WHEN AND HOW TO SEEK HELP

If you are concerned by any changes in the way you think or feel, this is enough reason to consult your doctor. There are numerous solutions to limiting anxious feelings, no matter how small they may seem. If it is big enough to impede your life or mental well-being at all, a doctor is likely to be able to share beneficial measures you can take. These could be as simple as introducing minor lifestyle changes that result in noticeable improvements in your mental health. Advice such as limiting your caffeine intake, adding an active element to your day, or learning new breathing techniques could ease some feelings of anxiety.

When the symptoms of anxiety escalate to the point that you are withdrawn from social activities; regularly experience feelings of dread, detachment, and irritability; or often feel physically panicked in situations, your doctor may suggest trying new medication. You may also be referred to a mental health professional, such as a trained therapist.

Considering speaking to someone you don't know about your anxiety can actually create mental hurdles, especially if you're already feeling more anxious than usual. After all, how are you meant to tell a stranger how you feel if you aren't entirely sure yourself? In most cases, the questions that a doctor will ask you about your thoughts will help you to process your feelings in ways you hadn't considered before. While this is new for you, health care professionals have the experience to know which type of treatment you are most likely to benefit from. Taking the first step and asking for help means you gain guidance, and the pressure to find the answers by yourself disappears.

Before your appointment, you may want to write down any questions you have, or new feelings you have experienced. This will give you reassurance that you won't forget to mention specific aspects of your anxiety or ask a question that comes to mind during the lead-up to the appointment.

Most importantly, try to be as open and honest in your appointment as you can. Time with doctors is often limited, but this time is crucial for them to gauge a true picture of you and your mental health.

At the end of the appointment you could be given some at-home methods to reduce anxiety, a prescription for anti-anxiety medication, or a suggestion for a specific therapy type. If you are unhappy with the advice given, you are within your rights to request a second opinion. Additionally, if you are only given medication, you can ask which talking therapy options are available to you.

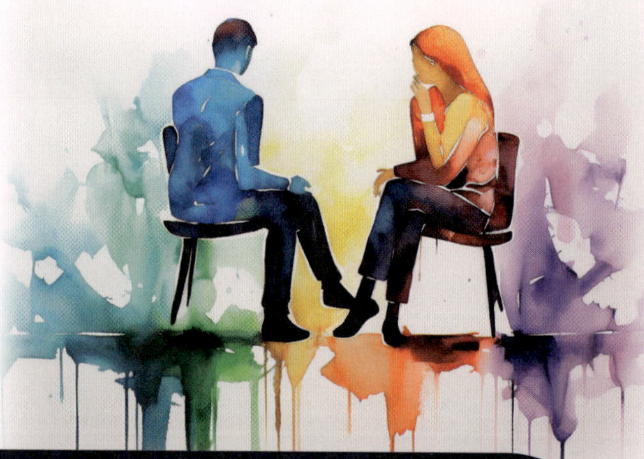

HYPNOTHERAPY

During a session, participants enter a state of mental relaxation and focus. While less research has been carried out on the effectiveness of hypnotherapy when compared to psychotherapy, it's thought that if someone can achieve a mental state of relaxation resembling sleep, the mind becomes more receptive. Depending on what a patient wishes to improve, suggestions will be made during the hypnosis that will reduce their anxiety in specific events. For example, if you had a phobia of animals and it was triggering anxiety symptoms, the hypnotherapy would focus on your perception of the animal. A therapist would target your subconscious to reprogram your thoughts surrounding the animal. In some instances, people have claimed that their mental response to their phobia changed after these sessions.

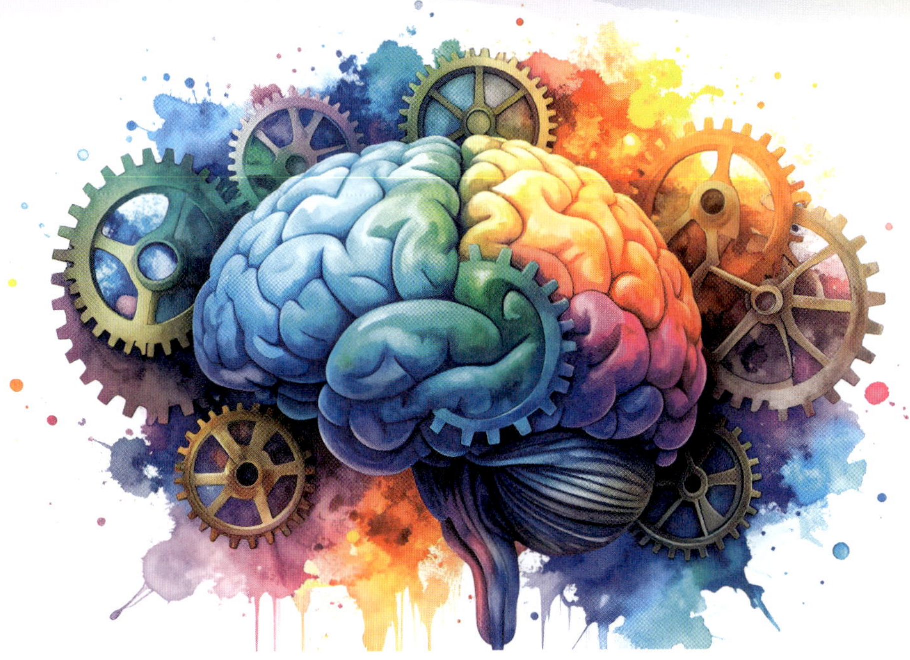

COGNITIVE BEHAVIORAL THERAPY

How does this treatment tackle negative thought cycles?

Sometimes it can be difficult to pinpoint the core cause of anxiety by yourself; it can actually be easier for someone else to detect unhelpful thoughts. The multitude of feelings that can arise are often overwhelming, but cognitive behavioral therapy (CBT) can help in some instances. CBT sessions involve speaking to a trained therapist to break down the negative thought cycles that result in anxiety, and tackle personal aspects. During these sessions, questions will be tailored toward finding an individual's problematic thoughts. Then, therapists will explore ways to deconstruct these thoughts and reconstruct them for a more positive outcome.

The main concept behind CBT is that situations, thoughts, emotions, physical feelings, and actions are all connected. The aim is to change a person's mental approach to daily situations to reduce the likelihood of events developing into anxious feelings.

CBT is one of the most successful treatments for generalized anxiety disorder, as it provides practical solutions to daily struggles. The treatment itself can involve between five and twenty one-hour sessions, but the mental techniques learned in this short space of time can assist you for life.

CBT is only effective if you are ready to be vulnerable and fully confront deep feelings. Underlying issues won't be explored in much depth, such as past events that may have caused anxiety, but CBT equips the patient to better navigate situations in the present.

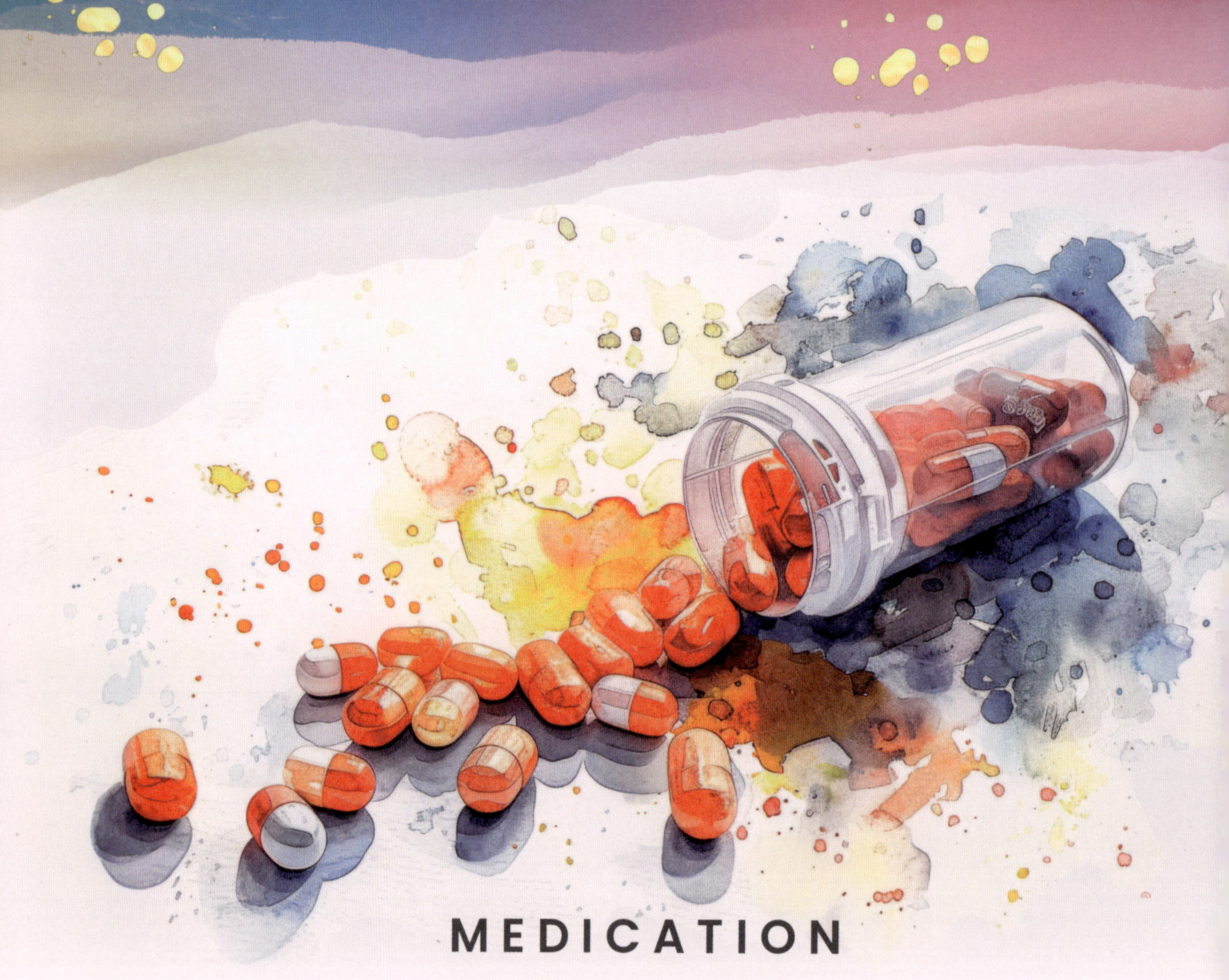

MEDICATION

To relieve the symptoms of anxiety, drugs can alter chemicals in the brain.

Medication for anxiety doesn't cure these disorders, but it can transform the life of someone suffering from one. By managing the symptoms of anxiety, medication helps a person to feel more like themselves and function better. There is a diverse selection of medication available, so you should consult your doctor to find the best option for you. You may need to test out more than one before finding the best solution for you.

Anti-anxiety medication usually works by increasing the mood-altering chemicals in the brain. For short-term treatment, a sedative called benzodiazepines can be taken to relax both the muscles and the mind. Because this medication is a sedative, it can cause drowsiness, and issues with balance or memory, so it should only be taken for the short period that it is prescribed for. There are different types of benzodiazepines for anxiety, but be warned: Xanax is deemed to be one of the more dangerous ones. Some people develop a dependence on Xanax, and sudden withdrawal from it can lead to lethal seizures. To avoid developing dependence on benzodiazepines, the dosage should be reduced gradually if this medication has been taken for two weeks or more.

Increasing the levels of serotonin in the body can be achieved through medication called selective serotonin reuptake inhibitors (SSRIs). Serotonin is a neurotransmitter that helps to regulate mood and anxiety, among other things. Dosage of SSRIs usually starts low and is built up to get the body used to the medication, because side effects differ between people. These include nausea, excessive sweating, and drowsiness.

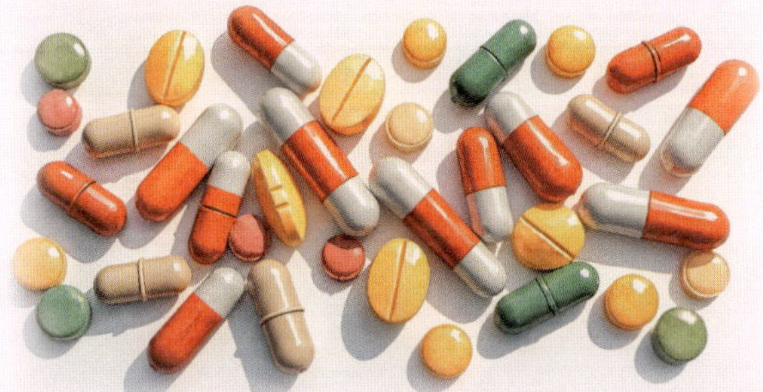

Some of the physical effects of anxiety are targeted with beta blockers, such as propranolol. This medication works to prevent event-related anxiety attacks, which are brought on in stressful situations. By blocking norepinephrine and epinephrine (adrenaline) from taking effect, this medication prevents reactions such as tightness in the chest and rapid heart rates.

EXPOSURE THERAPY

Exposure therapy is a technique that can be used to combat both generalized and social anxiety disorders that are focused around specific phobias. Psychologists aim to reduce the anxious feelings that emerge in individuals when faced with a phobia by subjecting them to their phobia. This might sound counterintuitive and damaging, but research shows that experiencing your biggest fear in a controlled environment reduces the negative responses felt when the situation is repeated elsewhere.

Exposure therapy doesn't have to involve real-life exposure, but it can. You could be asked to perform in front of an audience if you suffer from social anxiety, or instructed to interact with your phobia. Imaginal exposure, on the other hand, could be centered around a past traumatic event that causes anxiety attacks. Being asked to recall this negative experience can help someone to rethink the events and face their fear mentally.

By completing these tasks in a safe space, people find that they gain confidence around their phobia through better understanding and familiarity of it. Demonstrating that they are capable of navigating the situation shows them that they can do so again if they need to. In other instances, the negative associations they held with the object or activity they were exposed to, and the resulting anxiety, are reduced.

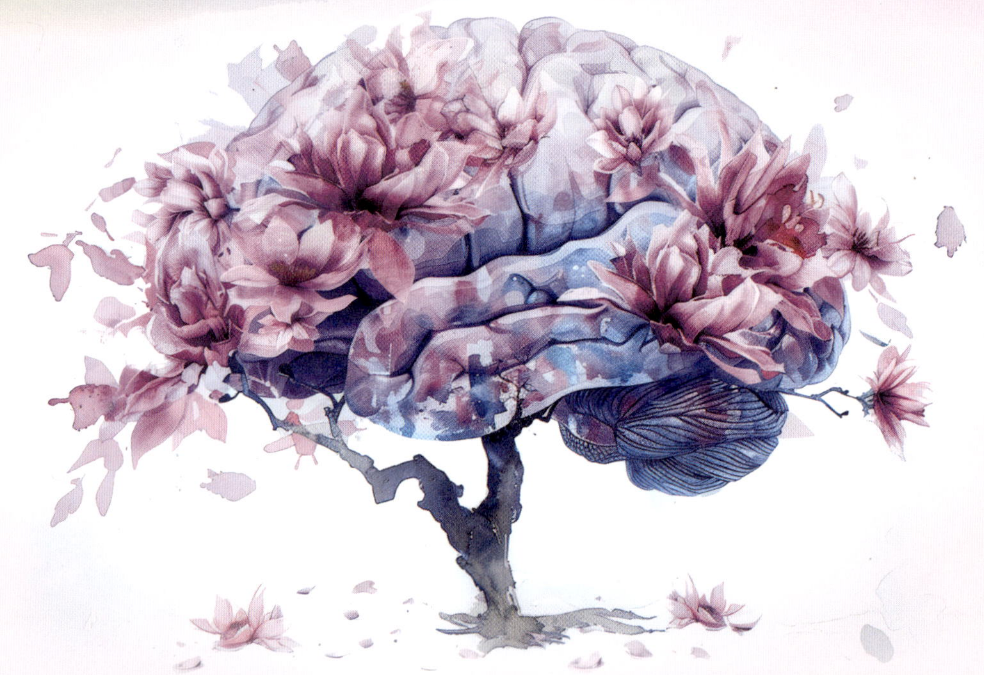

APPLIED RELAXATION THERAPY

These methods help you gain control of your body.

Relaxing may seem impossible during extreme anxiety, but learning relaxation techniques to reduce muscle tension and slow your breathing can help to reduce the intense sensations of this disorder. Knowing effective methods to regain control over your body can be life changing.

Applied relaxation therapy includes a wide array of mind-body exercises that aim to calm the body's fight-or-flight response. As everybody is different, it's worth testing out a few with a therapist to find the technique that best allows you to relax. However, relaxation might not work at all for some. By actively trying to stop the effects of anxiety when you are most distressed, you might send additional signals to your brain that you're in danger. If this happens, your body's uncontrolled defense response could increase or remain high. In this case it is best to use these techniques when you are not at your most distressed.

Some examples of techniques that you can try are slow diaphragmatic breathing and progressive muscle relaxation. To achieve deep breathing, inhale and exhale slowly, while avoiding lifting the shoulders. You should place one hand on your upper chest and the other below your rib cage. Focus on each breath, pushing only your lower hand outward. This strengthens the diaphragm and relaxes the body.

To feel the benefits of progressive muscle relaxation, tense any muscle for fifteen seconds. Then, release the muscle and count to thirty. When this works well, you should feel the sensation of relaxation pass through your body.

EYE MOVEMENT DESENSITIZATION AND REPROCESSING

There are conflicting opinions on the success of this relatively new method.

Research shows that eye movement desensitization and reprocessing (EMDR) can reduce feelings of anxiety when recalling a distressing past event. Many health care professionals believe more research needs to be conducted on this form of therapy, while others say they have witnessed its success.

The therapy involves the patient recalling their emotionally charged memories while focusing their eyes on the therapist's finger. As the individual speaks of the event, which is usually avoided due to anxiety, the theory is that they change how the memory is stored. Because they were focusing their attention on their eye movement, they feel more comfortable mentally revisiting this traumatic event.

While experts are unsure exactly how the results unfold, this method has reduced the intensity of psychological responses for many individuals when they later retrieve anxiety-inducing memories.

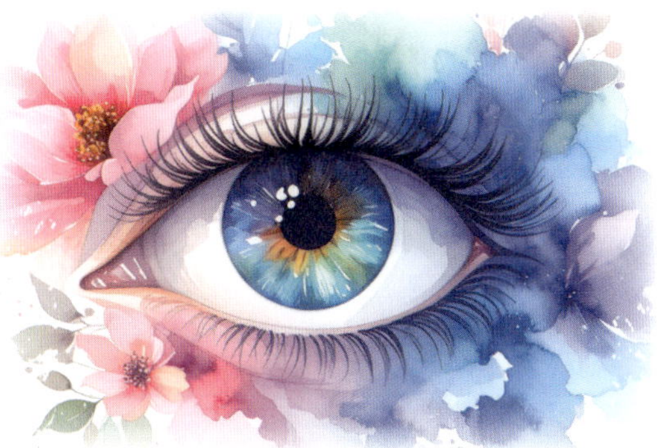

EXPOSURE AND RESPONSE PREVENTION

This is one of the most effective forms of treatment for people experiencing obsessive compulsive disorder (OCD). OCD is an anxiety disorder that causes recurring thoughts or repetitive behaviors that can't be controlled.

Exposure and response prevention (ERP) is a form of behavioral therapy that intentionally triggers a person's obsession and attempts to control it in a safe environment. For example, some people with OCD develop compulsive rituals. To an observer these may seem like small acts, but if the sufferer doesn't carry out the specific ritual, their anxiety builds. If somebody has an OCD ritual whereby they need to lock and unlock a door a certain number of times, they will be challenged to not do this in an ERP session. By asking them to walk through a door and refrain from locking it, they will need to work on controlling the resulting feelings. At first they may be overwhelmed with anxiety, but each time they are exposed to this situation, the anxiety can lessen.

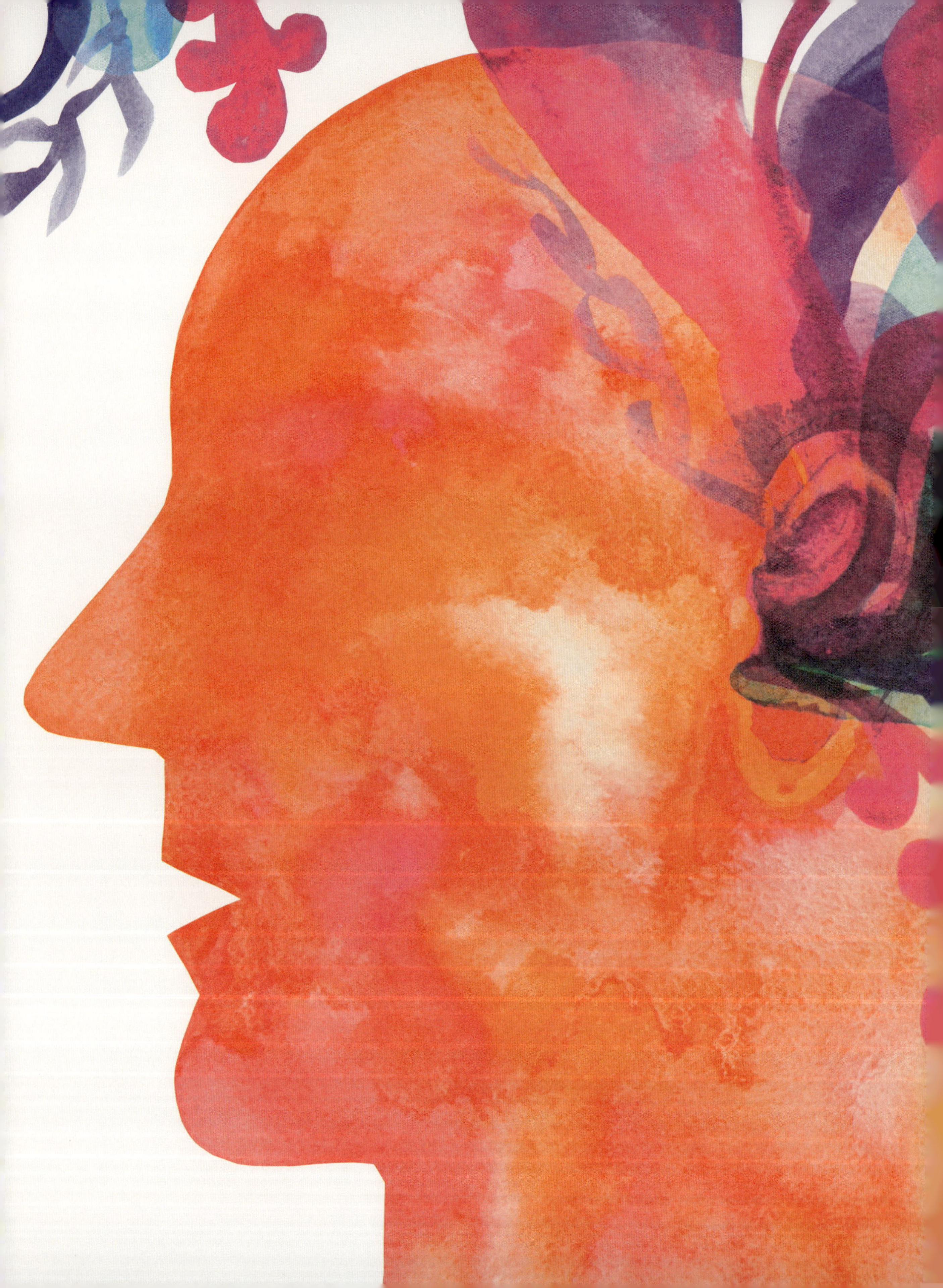

5-4-3-2-1 technique

Employing the five senses to return to the present.

During a panic attack, or when we can feel anxiety ramping up, the body and brain are locked into a feedback loop. Feelings of anxiety make the deep brain think it is in danger, which leads to it pumping out emergency hormones while getting the body ready to fight or flee. These elevated physical levels feed the physical sensations that accompany anxiety, making us more anxious, which leads to the deep brain pumping out even more emergency hormones. But all of this is going on inside us. There is no danger. Even if the anxiety trigger is something like a forthcoming event, the event hasn't happened yet—there is no need to panic. However, the deep part of the brain does not know this.

Future fear has translated into a panic attack in the present. If we can pull our focus back to the present, where in fact there is nothing dangerous, then the body can respond in turn. The 5-4-3-2-1 technique is a way of dissolving future fears into the immediate reality of our surroundings. To begin, as an immediate calming technique, slow the breath. Breathe in for a count of four and then out for a count of four. Repeat.

Keep this breathing pattern throughout the exercise, but the next time you breathe out, look around your surroundings and say out loud the names of five things you can see. They could be in the room with you (a chair, a bookcase) or outside, visible through a window (a tree, the sky). Then say the names of four things you can hear. They can be things loud or quiet, near or far. The point is to focus the attention in your ears at this point. The third step is to say three things you can feel. This could be the chair under you, the weight of clothes on your shoulder, or the breeze on your cheek. The fourth step is to name two things we can smell. If you don't have a particularly sensitive sense of smell, it might work to carry around something that has a distinctive odor to focus on when you need to employ the 5-4-3-2-1 technique—a bottle of perfume or a stick of gum, for example. The gum will come in useful for the final step: taste. It doesn't matter what you use to engage the sense of taste, but something pleasant will help to wind the exercise down calmly.

The 5-4-3-2-1 technique is a focused sensory technique to shift our focus away from the storm of internal thoughts and feelings of a panic attack to the world outside ourselves. The technique conveys the message to our autonomic nervous system through all five senses that everything really is all right and it can switch off its emergency response.

Draw five things you can See

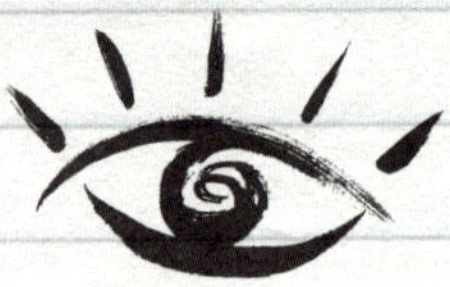

Draw four things you can Hear

Draw three things you can Feel

Draw two things you can Smell

Draw one thing you can Taste

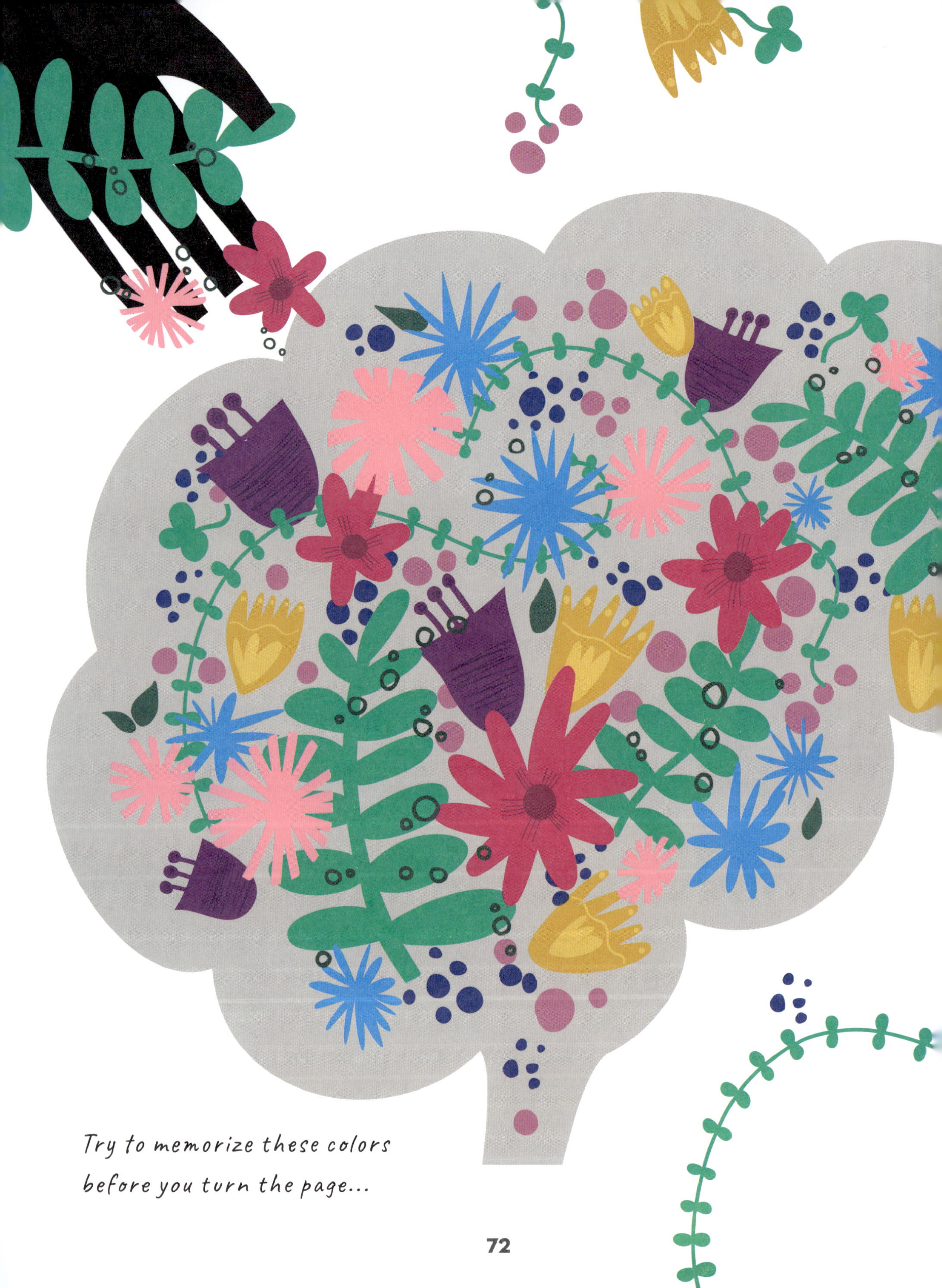

Try to memorize these colors
before you turn the page...

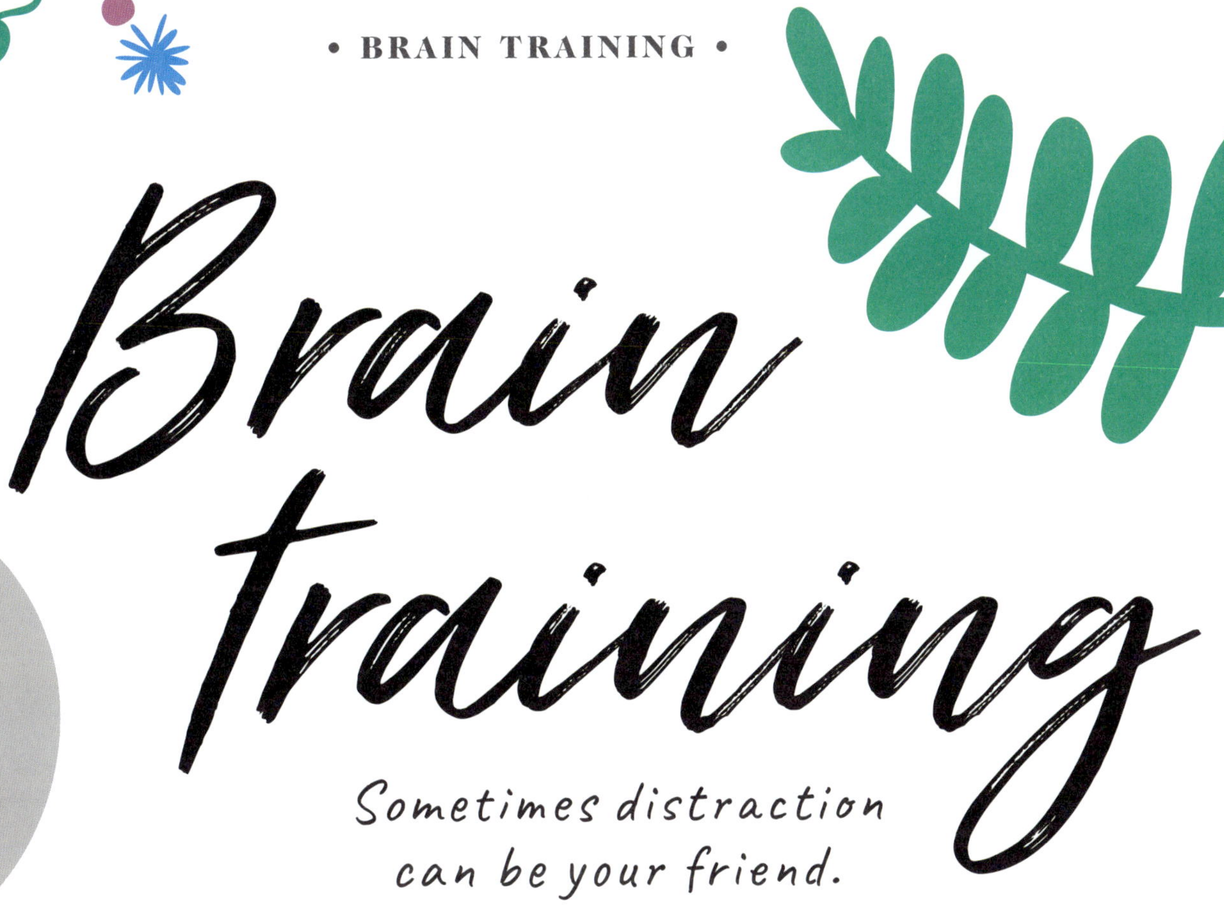

Brain Training

Sometimes distraction can be your friend.

The cycle of anxiety is perpetuated by distraction. While watching cat videos online before completing an important project may give you an instant release of tension, ultimately procrastination won't help you.

However, there are times when feelings of anxiety can become so overwhelming that simply relieving them becomes more important than anything else. In these cases, effective and nonharmful distraction techniques can be both helpful and necessary.

Among the most effective of these techniques are exercises that intensively use the most conscious part of our brains, the prefrontal cortex. This is also the part of the brain that is most prone to worry as a mental behavior, so finding something else for it to fixate on can allow the rest of the brain to slowly relax.

Any mental exercise that is demanding enough to require complete attention, but not too demanding to overtax a mind that is at its limits, is ideal. Many people find memory games useful. Visual thinkers might try to remember and visualize something familiar to them.

More physical mental games, from jigsaws to sudoku, can also be effective. However, as a general rule, high-intensity computer games should be avoided as these will increase stress.

Over the following pages, give your brain an escape from anxiety with various games, from visual challenges to anagrams.

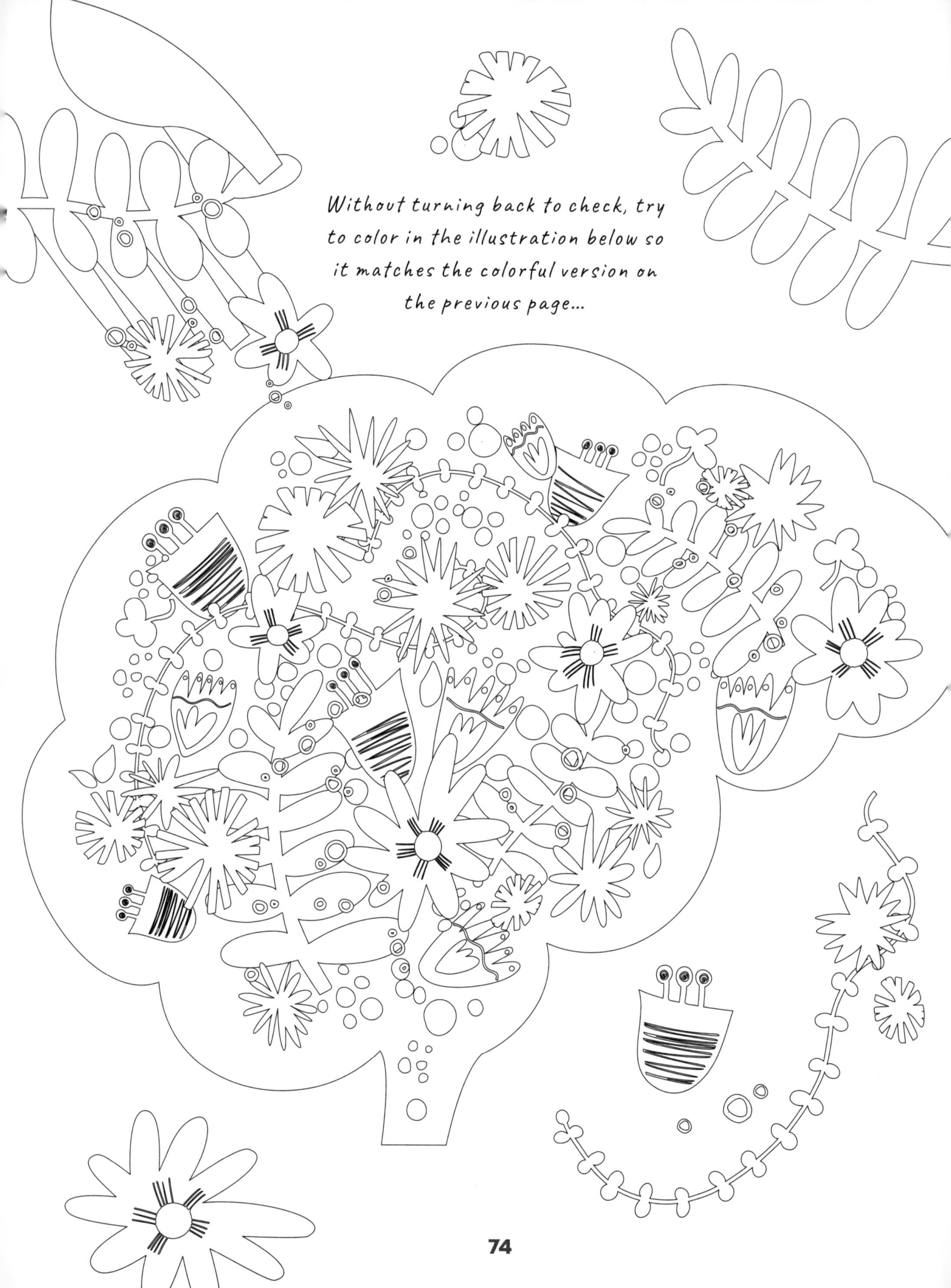
Without turning back to check, try to color in the illustration below so it matches the colorful version on the previous page...

SPOT THE DIFFERENCE

Can you find ten differences between the two pictures?

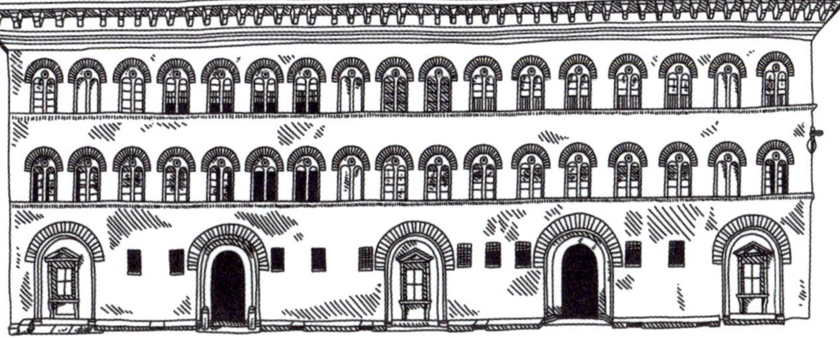

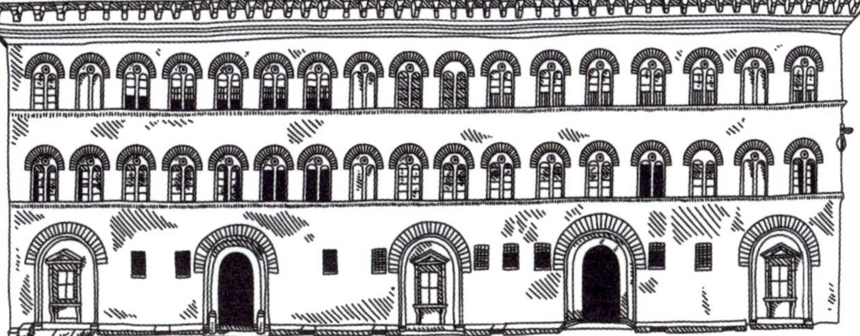

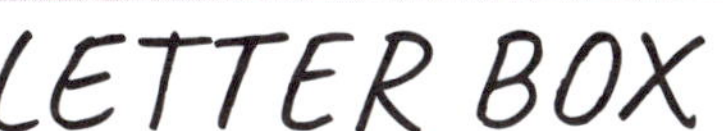

LETTER BOX

Cross out the letters that appear more than once. What word can you make with the remaining letters?

U	T	H	E	X	T	C
E	X	I	X	D	U	D
A	N	T	X	O	N	X
D	X	U	R	E	I	L
T	S	X	X	D	X	E

ANAGRAM

Rearrange the letters below to find a nine-letter word.

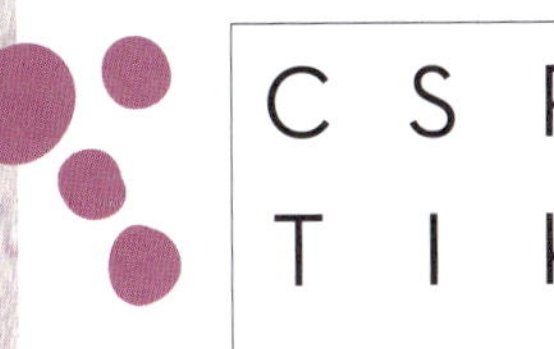

C	S	R
T	I	K
R	E	T

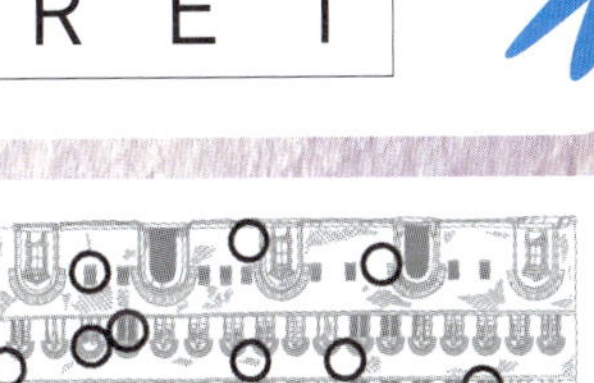

Mood Tracking

DISCOVER THE HIDDEN CUES AND NUANCES OF YOUR FEELINGS.

One of the key steps in freeing ourselves from the doom loop of anxiety is finding out what triggers anxious feelings. A therapist will often ask a client to keep a record of their feelings and the events of the day so that they can then together go back over the events of the week and try to discern if there is a pattern. Other people find it invaluable to write a journal of their feelings and experiences in order to better understand their responses to life. Both of these work very well with mood tracking.

In essence, mood tracking, or journaling, is keeping a diary. However, this is a diary of emotions. You keep track of your feelings throughout the day and week by making a record of them. In order to understand how the world affects your emotions, it's also necessary to note the main details of the day, too.

WRITE IT DOWN

As well as tracking your mood, try writing down what may affect your mood. Have you slept and eaten well? Have you exercised? Has anything negative happened?

The key part is simply keeping the record. Some people just write it down in a daily diary. Others write sticky notes, or record an account of the day's feelings on their phone. Nowadays, people also employ spreadsheets or apps.

Since it can be difficult to put feelings into words sometimes, particularly when we first attempt to do it, a mood chart might be helpful for identifying different emotions. Some idea of the level of the emotion is often useful, which can be done by writing next to the feeling an intensity scale from 1 to 10. With generalized anxiety disorder, a careful record of periods of heightened anxiety and panic attacks is particularly important.

Like keeping a diary, mood tracking is a very personal approach to dealing with anxiety, and while it is suitable for some people, it might not be for others.

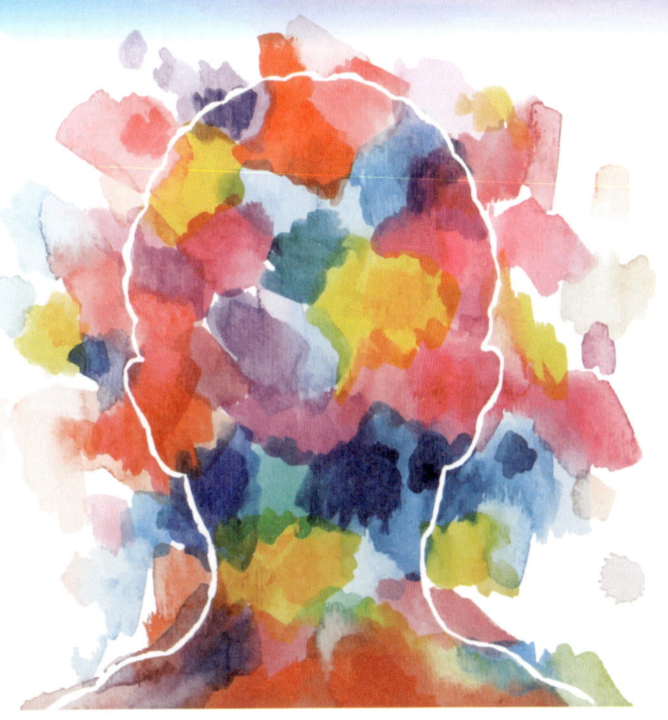

TODAY'S MOOD

	Calm	Happy	Sad	Angry	Disappointed	Worried	Scared	Frustrated
Mon								
Tues								
Wed								
Thurs								
Fri								
Sat								
Sun								

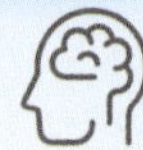

REFRAME NEGATIVE THOUGHTS

Cognitive distortions help to explain why we have unhelpful or negative thoughts, so the next step is being able to catch those thoughts and think about them in a different way. This is called "reframing." It isn't about ignoring your thoughts or pushing them away, but neither is it about being relentlessly positive.

First, you identify an unhelpful thought, then challenge it—is it accurate and based on fact, or is it something you have decided is true? Next, you try to come up with a more balanced or helpful thought to replace it. For example, "I did a terrible job on that piece of work, which proves I'm not capable of anything" could become "That wasn't my best work, but I know how I can improve and do a great job next time."

ALLOW TIME TO WORRY

Set aside a short period of time each day to think about your worries and give them space, but when the time's up, do something you enjoy and move on with your day.

List three negative thoughts you have identified recently.

1.

2.

3.

Take each of the negative thoughts you identified and think about how they make you feel, how you can reframe them, and whether that changes the way you feel.

Negative thought

....

....

How does it make you feel?

1 – 2 – 3 – 4 – 5 – 6 – 7 – 8 – 9 – 10

← Very calm — Neutral — Very anxious →

How could you reframe this thought?

....

....

How do you feel now?

1 – 2 – 3 – 4 – 5 – 6 – 7 – 8 – 9 – 10

← Very calm — Neutral — Very anxious →

Negative thought

....

....

How does it make you feel?

1 – 2 – 3 – 4 – 5 – 6 – 7 – 8 – 9 – 10

← Very calm — Neutral — Very anxious →

How could you reframe this thought?

....

....

How do you feel now?

1 – 2 – 3 – 4 – 5 – 6 – 7 – 8 – 9 – 10

← Very calm — Neutral — Very anxious →

Negative thought

....

....

How does it make you feel?

1 – 2 – 3 – 4 – 5 – 6 – 7 – 8 – 9 – 10

← Very calm — Neutral — Very anxious →

How could you reframe this thought?

....

....

How do you feel now?

1 – 2 – 3 – 4 – 5 – 6 – 7 – 8 – 9 – 10

← Very calm — Neutral — Very anxious →

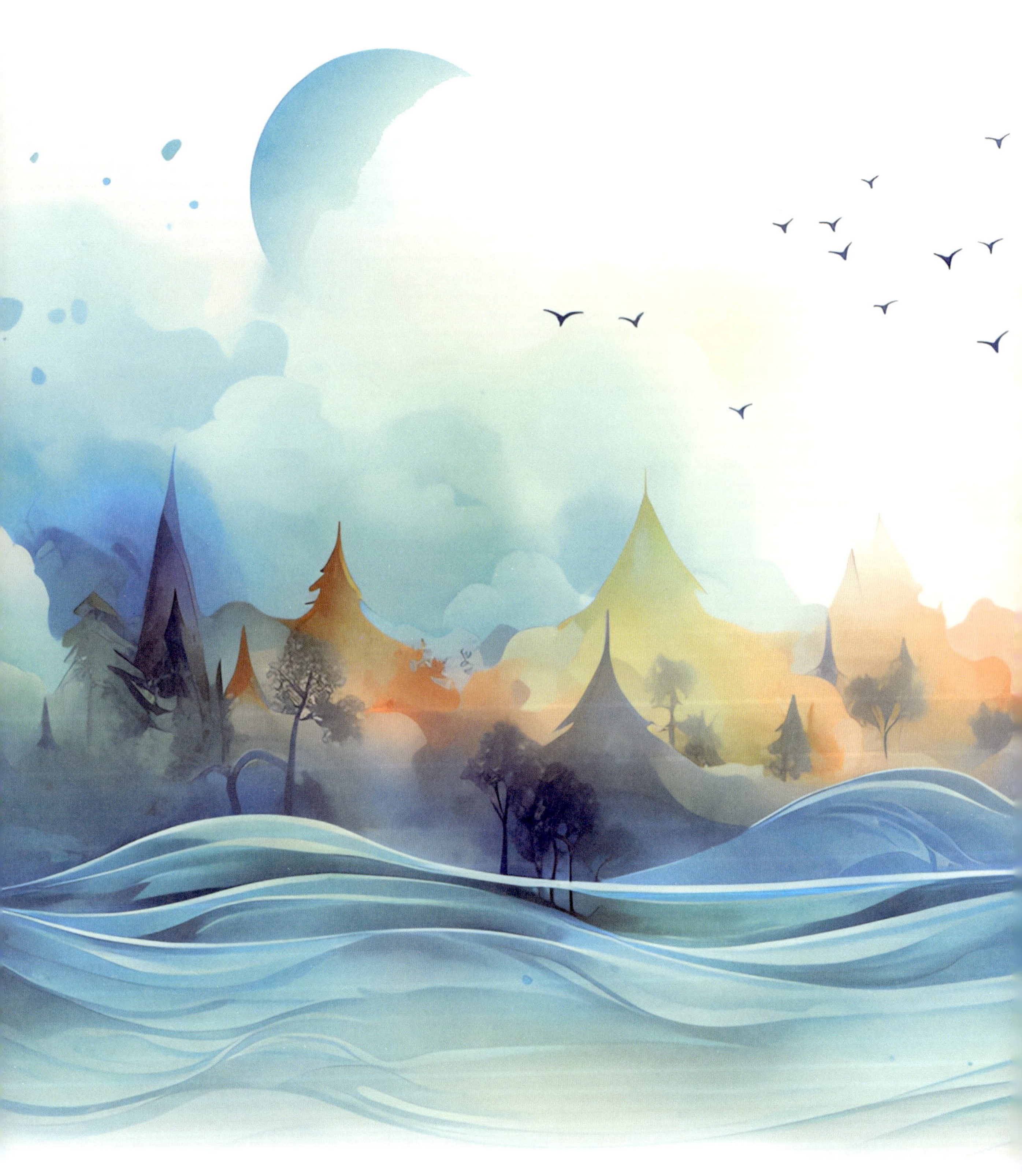

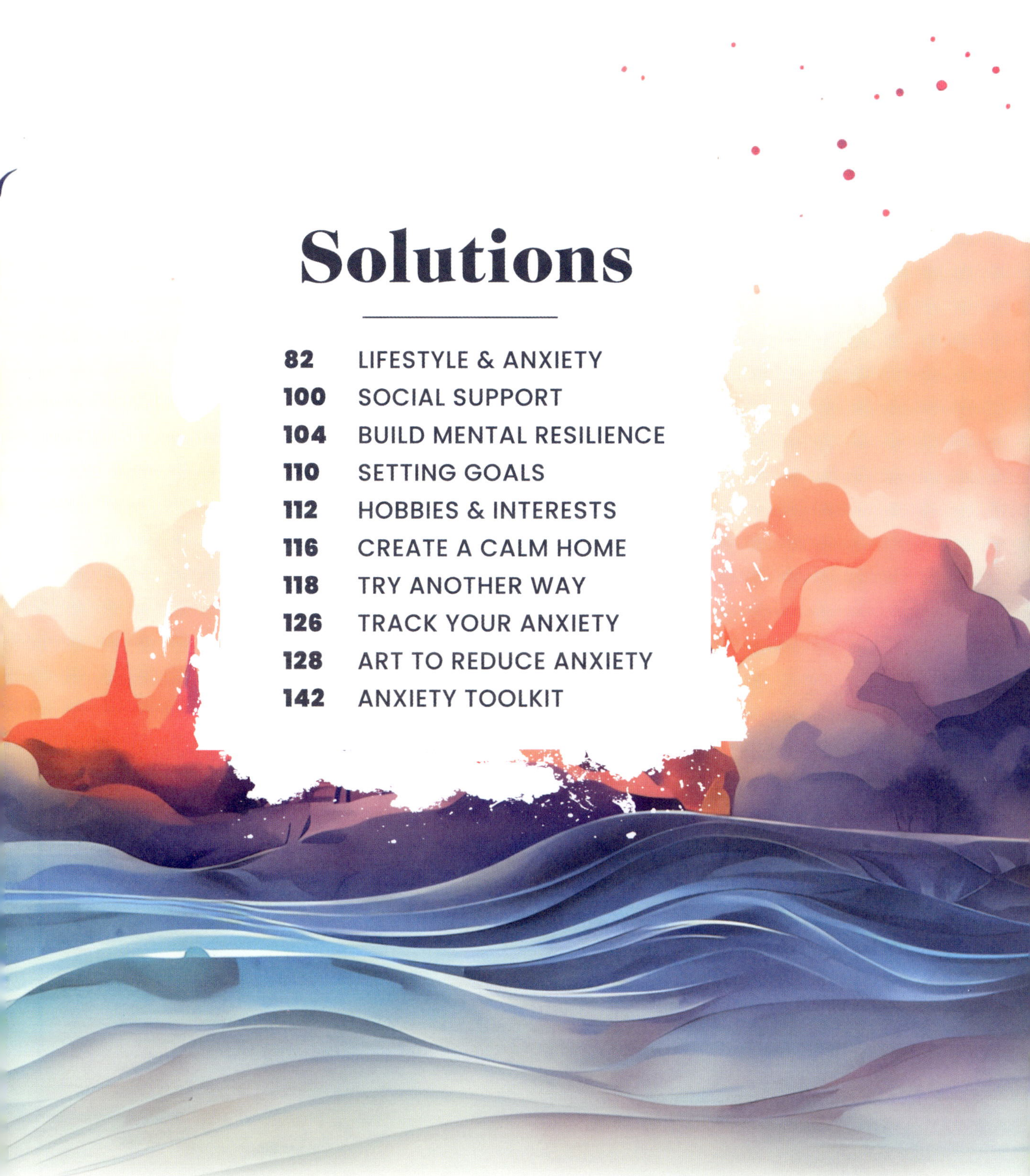

Solutions

Lifestyle & Anxiety

MAKING SMALL CHANGES IN YOUR DAILY LIFE CAN HELP YOU MANAGE YOUR ANXIETY.

Lifestyle choices can have a big impact on your anxiety, contributing directly to symptoms and making it harder to manage. If you have a poor work/life balance, eat a lot of processed foods on the go, have fitful sleep, or don't prioritize being active, these can all increase your anxiety. It's not uncommon, however, to have these lifestyle triggers—modern life is incredibly busy and often frantic, as we're all trying to juggle so many different roles. We have new pressures and stressors, such as social media, screen time, and long commutes. We also have access to vast quantities of information, which can make anxiety worse.

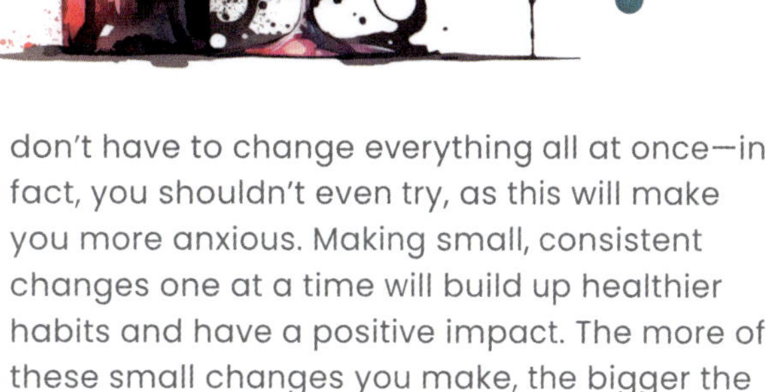

When you're feeling anxious or under stress, your body responds, preparing for "fight or flight," which over a long period of time can lead to physical health issues. When you combine this with unhealthy habits, such as a bad diet, lack of exercise, or drinking too much alcohol, your mind and body will find it harder to manage anxiety levels and symptoms. So while having that large glass of wine might make you feel less anxious in the moment, it won't help with long-term management of the condition.

When you have anxiety, however, it can feel overwhelming to make the necessary lifestyle changes. When you're already time-poor, a frozen meal feels so much simpler than cooking a healthy meal from scratch. When you're exhausted from a stressful day at work, going out for a run seems impossible. The key is not to take an "all or nothing" approach. You don't have to change everything all at once—in fact, you shouldn't even try, as this will make you more anxious. Making small, consistent changes one at a time will build up healthier habits and have a positive impact. The more of these small changes you make, the bigger the effect on your anxiety.

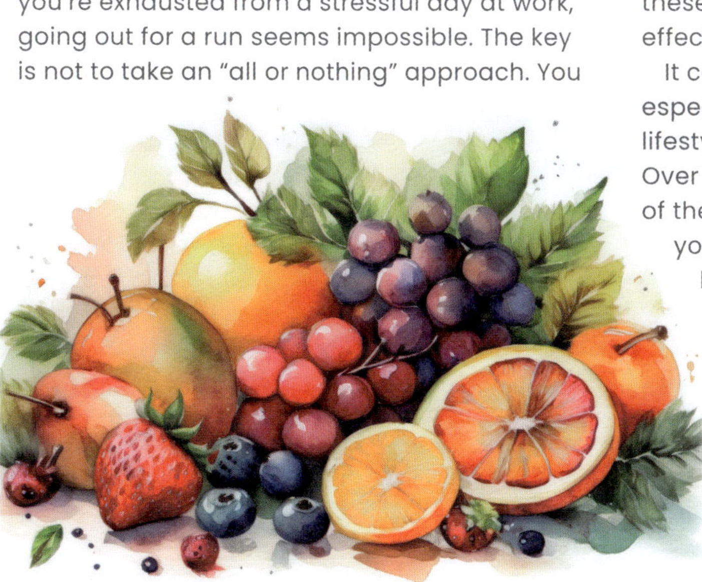

It can be hard to know where to start, especially if you feel like there are many lifestyle areas you need to improve upon. Over the next few pages, we'll look at some of the most common lifestyle interventions you can work on to manage your anxiety levels: nutrition, exercise, sleep, mindful movement, and stress. As you work through the prompts we've given you, you will hopefully identify which area or areas are impacting you the most to help you decide where to begin.

EATING TO EASE ANXIETY

Feeling stressed and anxious can lead to appetite changes, like nausea and skipping meals, to stress snacking salty and sugary foods and binge eating. It can be hard to consider your daily diet when you are struggling with work or life-related stress, but what we eat has a major effect on our emotions. For example, have you ever felt '"hangry"—hungry and angry at the same time? This feeling is caused by low blood sugar. When your blood sugar levels drop, it can cause irritability, depression, and tiredness. Thankfully, by being a little bit mindful over what foods you pick, you can help combat hanger and help your body fight negative feelings in general—and it's easier than you might think!

CONSIDER YOUR CARBS

Don't skip your carbs, no matter what the advice in magazines or on social media might say, as they are an essential source of energy. Keep your blood sugar levels steady by selecting foods that release energy in your body slowly. Brown rice and pasta, whole-grain bread and cereal, and nuts and seeds are all fantastic options. Try switching from white bread, pasta, and rice to the brown alternatives and see if you notice a difference.

HEALTHY HYDRATION!

What you drink is just as important as the foods you consume. When we are dehydrated, it becomes harder to think clearly and make decisions. It also affects our ability to concentrate.

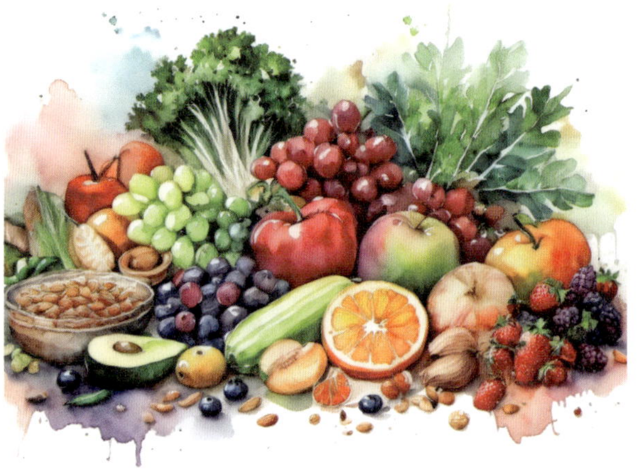

Water is always the best option for rehydration. Caffeine, a stimulant found in energy drinks, tea, coffee, soda, and chocolate (among other things), can often give you a burst of energy, but it can also dehydrate you and if it's not consumed in moderation, it can cause headaches, depression, anxiety, and sleep disturbance, especially if you drink it late in the day. Avoid having more than a couple of servings of tea, coffee, or soda in one day.

GET FRUITY!

Fruit and vegetables contain a wide range of vitamins, minerals, and nutrients that can help with both your physical and your mental health. Many contain vitamin C, which is vital to maintaining healthy brain function and essential for overall good health. Even dried, canned, or frozen fruit and vegetables can count toward your five a day.

Fruit juices and smoothies might seem healthy, but they can often contain high levels of hidden sugars. Studies have also shown that when you blend fruit, it loses some of the fiber that helps slow down the body's conversion of food sugars to blood sugars, meaning smoothies provide a shorter boost of energy than if you consumed the fruit in its natural state. However, if you struggle to get enough fruit and vegetables into your diet, making one smoothie at home for a yummy breakfast boost is still a good idea.

POSITIVE PROTEINS

Proteins are another essential. They contain chemicals called amino acids, and your brain needs these to produce neurotransmitters. These are the chemicals that get the nerve cells throughout your body to communicate, and they enable the brain to perform several key tasks. You can find good sources of protein in many foods like beans, lentils, soy products, milk, fish, eggs, nuts and seeds, lean meat, and cheese. Fatty acids like omega-3 and omega-6, which are found in oily fish, seeds, nuts, and avocados, are another critical ingredient for a healthy brain and can adequately regulate your feelings and emotions.

MUST-HAVE MINERALS

When it comes to calming your nervous system and managing stress responses, magnesium is a must. Magnesium is also helpful for females, as it can help with premenstrual syndrome.

There are also many vitamins that play an important part in reducing stress. Vitamin D and B vitamins, especially vitamin B12, vitamin B6, folate, and iron each offer something in the battle to keep anxiety at bay. These minerals particularly benefit females, as you can lose large amounts of iron and other vitamins when you menstruate, causing you to feel exhausted. Low iron is also directly linked to feelings of depression and anxiety, and having low energy levels can lead to feeling overwhelmed and being unable to manage your feelings.

Many vitamins and minerals can be taken as a supplement, but we advise first speaking with a health-care provider to see what vitamins you might benefit from and which ones you might be lacking. Vegetarians and vegans can find it more difficult to consume enough B vitamins and vitamin D, as they are mostly found in animal-based foods. So if you are following a vegan diet you will need to ensure you add foods fortified with these vitamins to your diet.

MINERALS FOR MENTAL HEALTH

MAGNESIUM	VITAMIN D	B VITAMINS	L-THEANINE	IRON	ZINC	CALCIUM
Found in:	**Found in:**	**Found in:**	**Found in:**	**Found in:**	**Found in:**	**Found in:**
Dark chocolate Spinach Whole wheat Almonds Cashews Black beans	Oily fish Sunlight—so make sure you find time to go out and soak up some rays!	Leafy green vegetables Eggs Mushrooms Nuts Chicken Peas	Green and black tea	Red meat Shellfish Spinach Legumes (kidney beans, edamame beans, and chickpeas) Mushrooms Quinoa	Shellfish Red meat Eggs Pomegranate Lentils Pumpkin seeds	Milk Cheese Salmon Kale Soybeans

NUTRITION TRACKER

When you feel anxious, it's easy to develop poor eating habits—whether that's skipping meals or eating more often than usual. However, making changes to your nutrition can help to ease the effects of anxiety. Focus on foods like fruits and vegetables, whole grains, and lean protein while limiting ultraprocessed, high-sugar, and high-fat foods. Think about variety and diversity, eating your "five a day," and opting for a mix of different colors on your plate. There is some evidence to prove that looking after your gut health can improve anxiety symptoms, so add in probiotics and fermented foods like yogurt, kimchi, and kefir.

Eat regularly, aiming for three balanced meals a day. Drink plenty of water as well, which can help to boost your energy and mood, and limit caffeinated drinks—caffeine can trigger anxiety symptoms in some people. Take this opportunity to review your current dietary habits and commit to some long-term goals.

"There is some evidence to prove that looking after your gut health can improve anxiety symptoms"

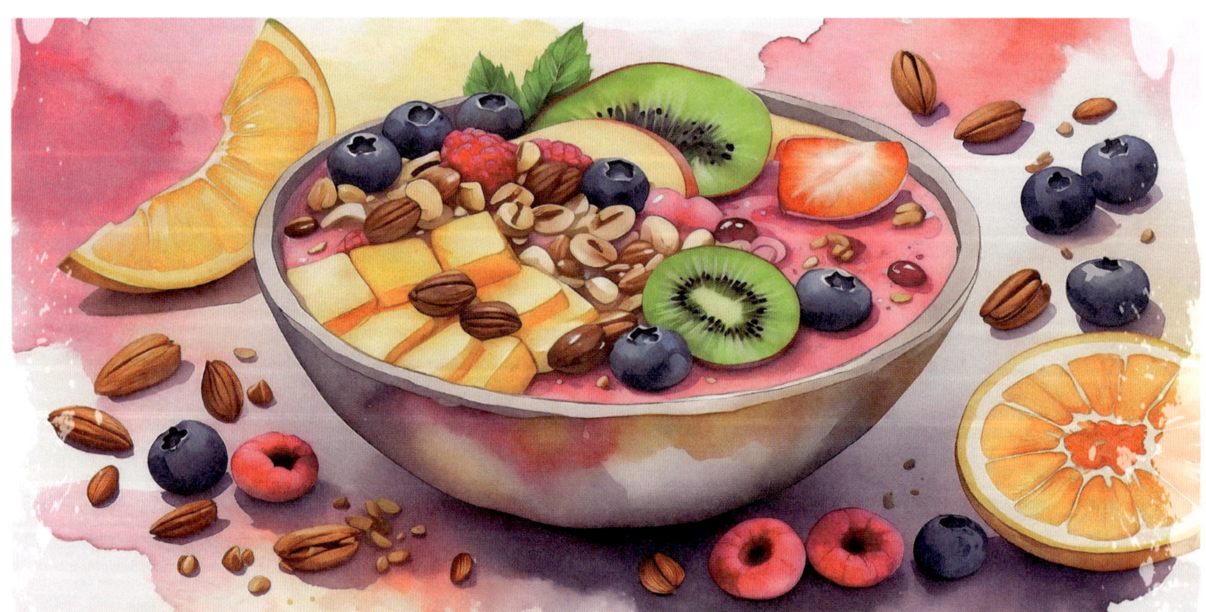

Track your food and drink intake honestly for the next three days— this can help you to identify any patterns or areas you can improve on.

DAY ONE	DAY TWO	DAY THREE
Breakfast	Breakfast	Breakfast
Lunch	Lunch	Lunch
Dinner	Dinner	Dinner
Snacks	Snacks	Snacks
Drinks	Drinks	Drinks

Did you notice any triggers that impacted your dietary choices? For example, some people find they eat more sugary foods when they're faced with a stressful situation.

What changes would you like to make to your overall diet? Use this space to outline any nutritional goals.

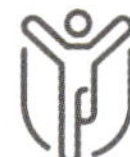

MOVE FOR YOUR MIND

Give your body a workout to help clear your mind, boost your brain, and even induce sleep!

Exercising can be a great way to help you cope with feelings of anxiety. Whether you do it alone, with a friend, or in a group, getting your heart pumping spells good news for your mental health. This is because physical activity releases endorphins—hormones that are linked to pleasure, pain relief, stress reduction, and an enhanced sense of well-being. Moving your body also decreases muscle tension, which in itself lowers an overall feeling of anxiety. Plus, when your heart rate increases during more vigorous aerobic exercise, it triggers a change in brain chemistry to boost the levels of several anti-anxiety chemicals, such as serotonin. On top of this, it also gives your mind a chance to focus on something that isn't the cause of your concern and divert your energy into something productive. Ideally, just one hour every day should be spent doing some form of movement. If you aren't a team sports type of person, here are a few examples of healthy activities that will benefit you.

TACKLE ANXIETY

Try out a combat sport to boost your confidence, courage, and self-esteem, as well as blasting away everyday stress and pent-up frustrations!

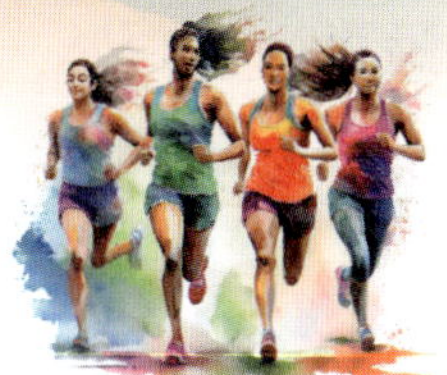

RUNNING

Running is a tried and tested way to clear your mind and stop you from focusing on what is stressing you out, which in turn reduces your stress levels. It is also an easy way to trigger your body to release mood-boosting chemicals and give you an increased feeling of happiness. However, if you aren't naturally attuned to it, it can be tough to get going, so begin slowly, easing yourself into it.

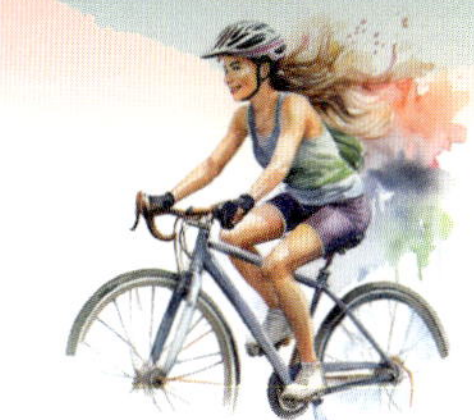

CYCLING

Just like running, cycling can help you get your heart rate up and also get you outside into the fresh air; however, it benefits from having a lower impact on your knees and ankles. Whether you just jump on your bike and take it for a spin around the park or devote yourself to a spin class, cycling is a great way to take your mind off your worries and get your heart pumping so you feel that all-important high!

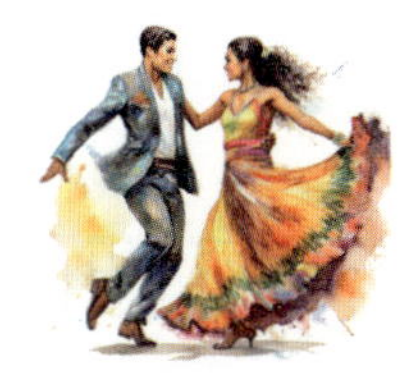

DANCING

Okay, so this might not be your first thought when embarking on some exercise, but you can do it at home or in an outside space. You could even join a group and make new friends. It's creative, expressive, fun, and challenges your brain. It raises the heart rate and focusing on a routine provides distraction from your worries, making it a great physical and mental workout!

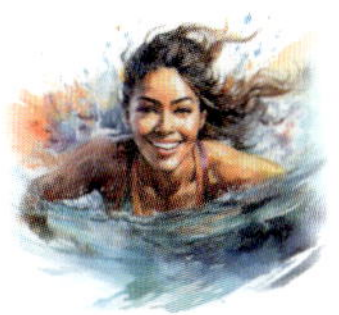

SWIMMING

Swimming is excellent for helping you to breathe deeply, calming the nervous system. Water itself has a soothing effect on the mind, and while swimming is a gentle, low-impact exercise—making it ideal if you suffer from any injuries or mobility issues—it still improves fitness levels, aids flexibility, and helps to release those essential happy hormones.

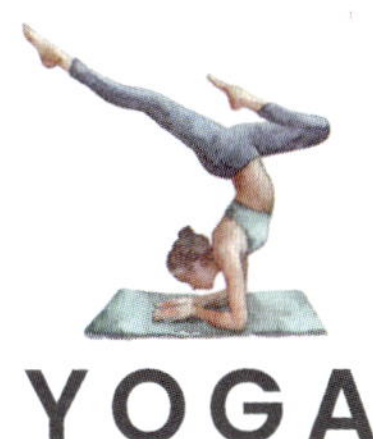

YOGA

Yoga combines controlled breathing with meditation and cardiovascular exercises to boost and improve your physical health and mental clarity. You can join a group or do it at home. There are numerous online sessions and videos, so you can choose which exercises suit you (plus nobody will know if you have fallen asleep).

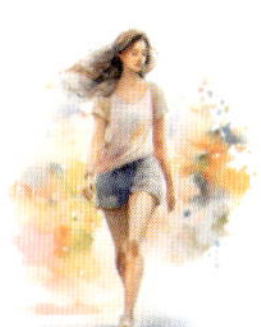

WALKING

Just getting out into the fresh air can be hugely beneficial. Walking (or hiking) increases blood flow and circulation, calming the nervous system, and reducing stress. Just twenty minutes a day can drastically improve your physical and mental health. Breathe deeply and observe the nature and environment around you—this can be a mood booster in itself!

TRACK YOUR EXERCISE

One of the most powerful things you can do to relieve the symptoms of anxiety is exercise. Being physically active can help to lower your stress levels, improve your mood, boost self-esteem, and help with sleep. Remember, all movement matters, so you don't have to be lifting weights in the gym every day or training for a running race, unless that's what you want to do.

Identify the kind of exercise you enjoy, whether that's dancing in your kitchen, going for long walks, or playing team sports. Once you've figured out what movement it is that you enjoy, you need to prioritize it and make sure you schedule it into your week. Start to think of it as a nonnegotiable appointment and a commitment to looking after your own needs.

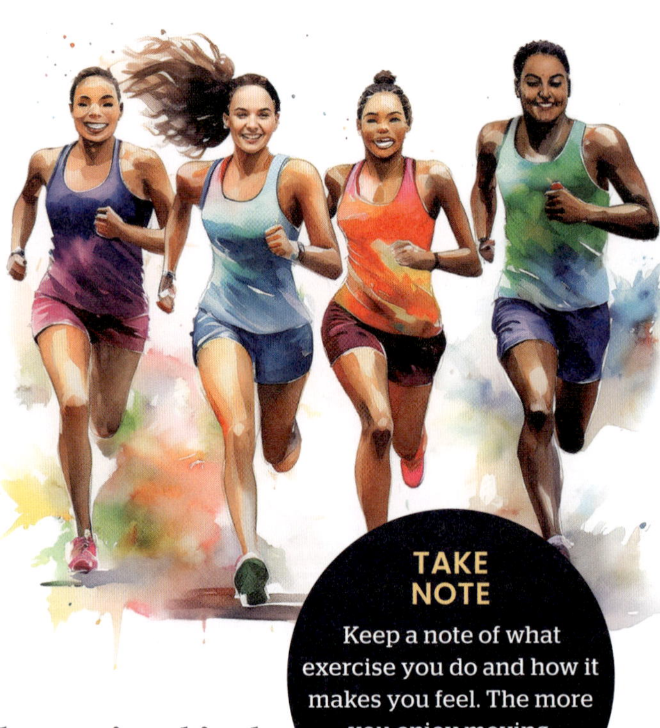

TAKE NOTE

Keep a note of what exercise you do and how it makes you feel. The more you enjoy moving, the more benefit you'll get.

What kind of exercise do you enjoy or have enjoyed in the past? This can be anything that gets your heart rate up, so don't be limited by traditional exercise concepts.

How are you going to make time to fit exercise into your week? Be realistic, but also set aside enough time for exercise.

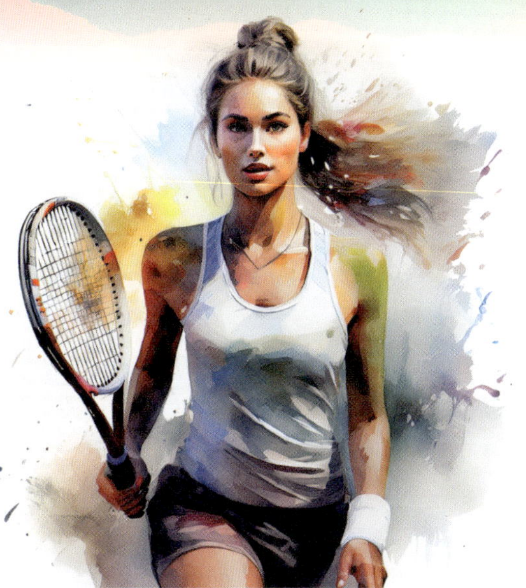

YOGA POSES TO TRY

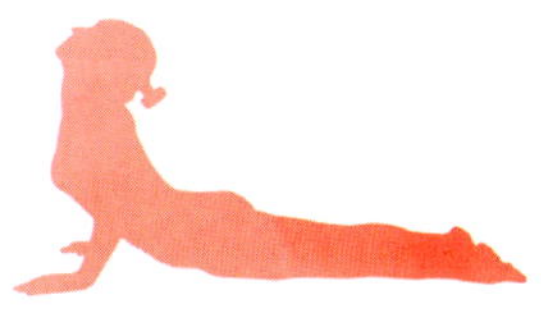

COBRA

Lie on your stomach, legs straight out behind you, hands under your shoulders. Lift your head and shoulders off the floor, looking up.

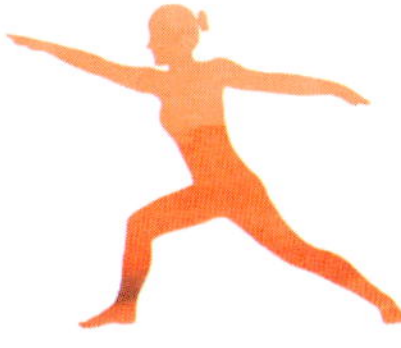

WARRIOR II

Stand feet wide apart. Turn your right foot 90 degrees, bending your knee. Extend your arms out to the sides, then hold the breath.

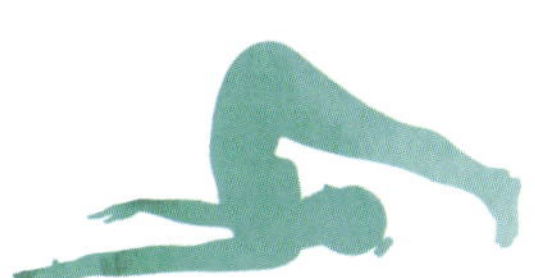

PLOW POSE

Lying down, stretch your legs back over your head, keeping your arms at your side. Hold and breathe to stretch out the spine.

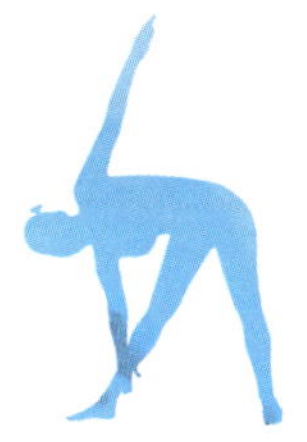

TRIANGLE

Stand with your feet apart. Turn your right foot 90 degrees. Extend your right hand downward and your left hand up. Breathe deeply.

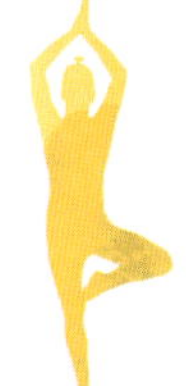

STANDING TREE

Stand on one leg and bring your other leg up to rest on your inner calf or thigh. Bring your hands together above your head.

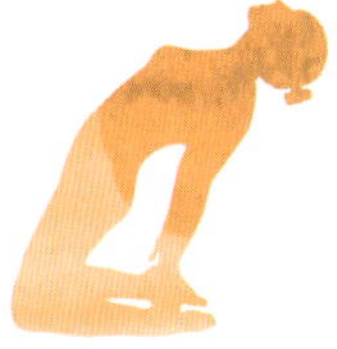

CAMEL POSE

Kneel on the floor. Then lean backward, breathing in until your hands reach your heels. Hold the pose, then sit back up.

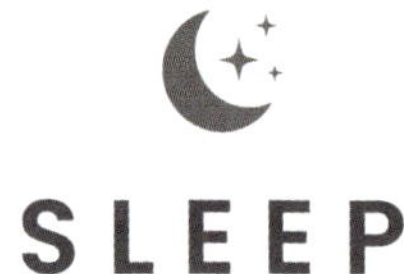

SLEEP

Problems with sleep and anxiety go hand in hand. If you're worrying a lot, this can make it difficult to go to sleep and stay asleep. However, if you're not getting enough sleep, this can make symptoms worse, and you can end up in a vicious cycle. We need enough good-quality sleep every night to help repair our internal systems, both physically and mentally. This starts with creating good sleep habits and an optimal sleeping environment.

Aim to go to bed and get up at roughly the same time every day. Avoid caffeine and alcohol in the evenings, so you're not overly stimulated. Switch off screens and devices at least an hour before bedtime and try something offline like reading or doing a puzzle to help you relax. Make sure your bedroom is dark and quiet. Think about your current sleep habits and if there are any improvements that you can make to ensure you get your rest.

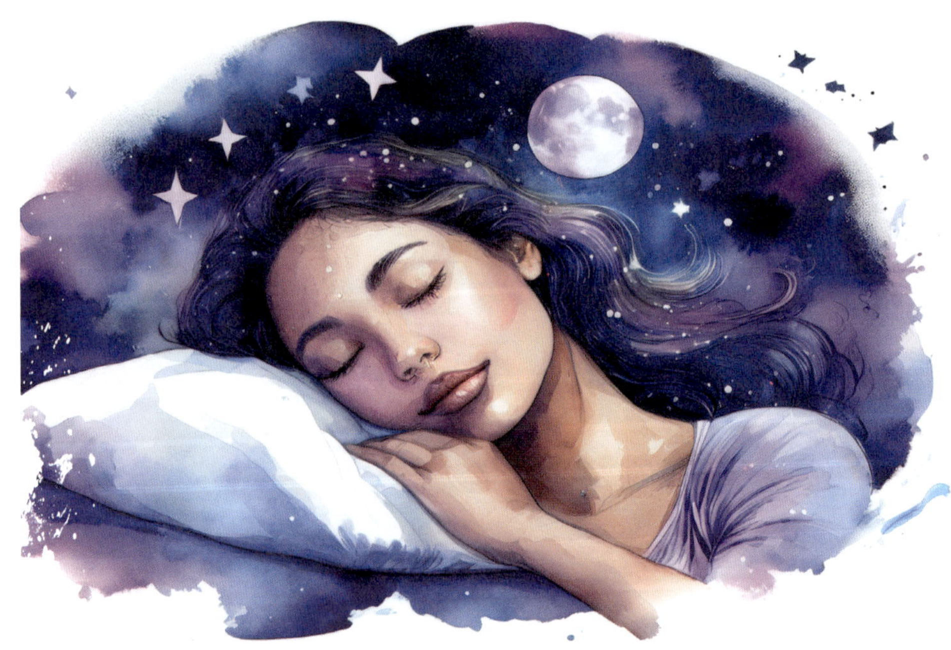

Log the details of a typical night's sleep using the prompts below, to give an overall picture of your current sleep habits.

Alcohol consumed

YES / NO

Time of last alcoholic drink

Caffeine consumed

YES / NO

Time of last caffeinated drink

Exercised today

YES / NO

Time went to bed

Time went to sleep

Number of times awoke in the night

Wake-up time

How I felt when waking up

What is impacting your sleep most?

What could you do differently to improve your sleep quality?

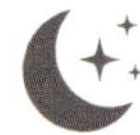

TOO STRESSED TO SLEEP

Need help to get some much-needed rest during times of stress? Here's how.

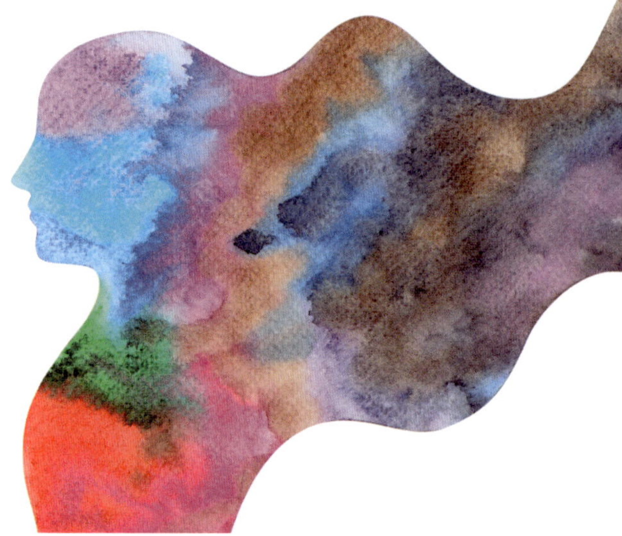

CUT THE CAFFEINE EARLIER

"Most of us are aware that drinking a cup of coffee straight before bed is likely to keep us up at night, but many underestimate the effect that our caffeine intake throughout the day could be having on our sleep habits," says Dr. Sarah Jarvis. "If you're regularly struggling to nod off, try cutting caffeine out completely from lunchtime onwards to see if it has a positive effect on your sleeping habits."

DON'T USE YOUR PHONE ON THE TOILET

Always scrolling? "When standing in a queue, we turn to our smartphones, and some people don't even go to the toilet without theirs," says Dr. Nerina Ramlakhan. "This leaves no time for your body and mind to properly process things in our lives, so our thoughts reappear and keep the mind going, which can be a particular problem when we try to go to sleep." If you're guilty, then schedule in smartphone downtime during the day.

EASE OFF THE BOOZE

"It can be tempting to have a drink or two to 'unwind' before bed, especially if you're feeling stressed—but, while alcohol may help you get off to sleep, it can lead to disrupted sleep," says Dr. Jarvis. "You're also more likely to experience rebound anxiety the next morning."

HAVE A SET WIND-DOWN ROUTINE

"If you have to work in the evening, stop at least an hour before you need to get to bed," says medical nutritionist Dr. Naomi Beinart. "Write down your to-do list for the next day. Then do anything that relaxes you, such as having a bath and then reading for twenty minutes. Having a set wind-down routine helps your mind and body to let go of the day and prepare for sleep."

EXERCISE AT THE RIGHT TIME

"Those who do a cardio workout (such as swimming or jogging) at 7:00 a.m. sleep longer, fall into deeper sleep cycles, and spend 75 percent more time in reparative slumber than those who work out later in the day," says Dr. Jarvis. "Cardio workouts also elevate the body's temperature, so exercise at least three hours before bedtime in order to avoid a disrupted sleep schedule."

AND BREATHE...

"Forms of meditation have been proven to help relax the body and mind," says Neil Robinson, chief sleep officer at Sealy UK. "Slowly inhaling and exhaling will help to calm your nervous system, lower your heart rate, and lead to you feeling relaxed ahead of your bedtime."

Try this recommended breathing exercise to relax your mind and body and switch off:

1. Lie in bed, arms away from your sides, palms facing up.
2. Breathe deeply in through your nose, counting steadily from one to five (or as far as you can comfortably).
3. Without pausing, breathe out gently through your mouth, counting to five. Keep going for about three to five minutes.

CREATE A HAVEN IN THE BEDROOM

Bedroom full of clutter? It could be adding unnecessary stress. "Make your bed a place you enjoy spending time in, rather than dread," says Robinson. "A comfortable healthy sleeping environment will promote deep and restful sleep."

HERBAL HELPERS

Need to de-stress? Try these natural remedies:

- Valerian root can help aid anxious thoughts and improve sleep quality.
- Marine magnesium, which is derived from seawater, can calm the nervous system.

STOP STRESSING ABOUT THE TIME

Do you look at the clock when you wake in the night? It could be doing you more harm than you realize. This is because over-measurement of sleep, especially using tracking devices, is causing a new disorder called orthosomnia. "This is where you're unhealthily preoccupied with how much sleep you are or aren't getting," says Dr. Ramlakhan. The solution? Distract yourself. "It's very easy to start counting down the hours until you need to be up in the morning and getting stressed as a result," says Dr. Jarvis. "Cover up the clocks, get up, and do something else in another room, such as reading a book. Once you start feeling more relaxed you can try going back to bed—sometimes a change of scene is enough to help you nod off."

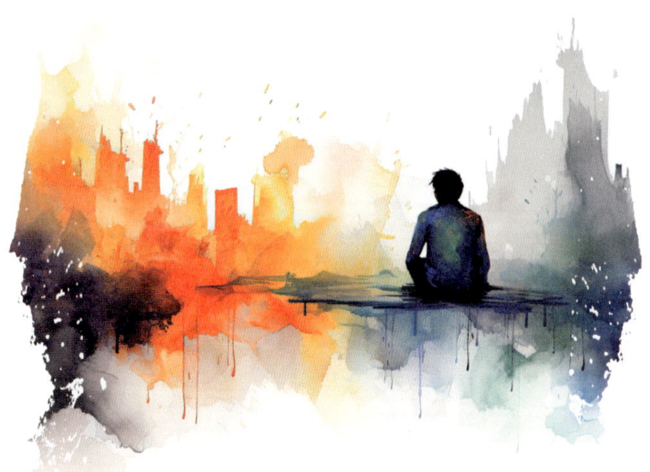

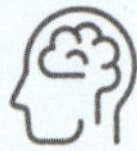

MINDFUL MOVEMENT

Mindfulness is a practice that helps you to tap into the connection between mind and body, and can help to reduce stress and ease anxiety. By combining mindfulness and movement, you can become more aware of your body, lift your mood, and feel more energetic. When you move mindfully, it's about being focused on the present moment, not worrying about the future or ruminating on the past. This might mean concentrating on your breath as it flows in and out, feeling the ground beneath your feet, or noticing the natural world around you.

If your mind wanders, gently ease it back to the here and now. Mindful movement includes things like walking outside, and gentle practices like yoga or Pilates, where you need to focus on your movements and breath to get the most out of them. Give it a go by trying our simple exercise on the opposite page.

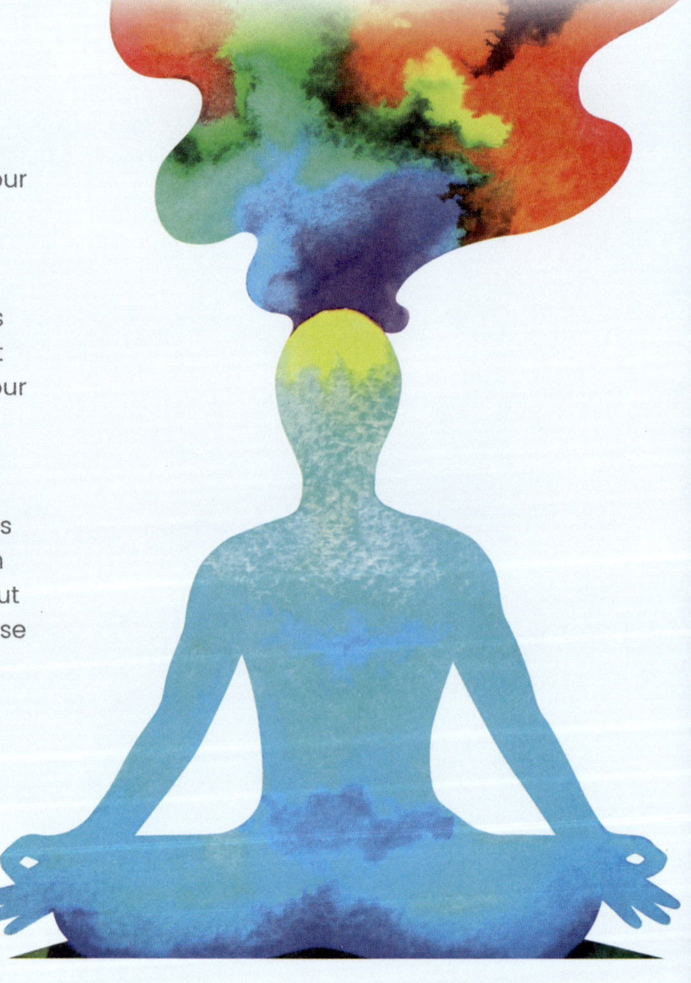

"When you move mindfully, it's about being focused on the present moment"

Go for a walk with the intention to be mindful of your surroundings. Pay attention to how your body feels, how the ground feels beneath your feet, what you can see around you, what you can hear around you, and so on. When you get back, write down your observations here.

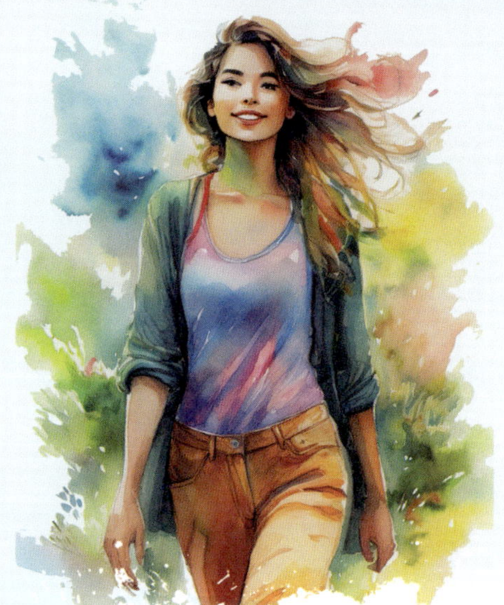

How did the mindful walk make you feel? Did you enjoy it?

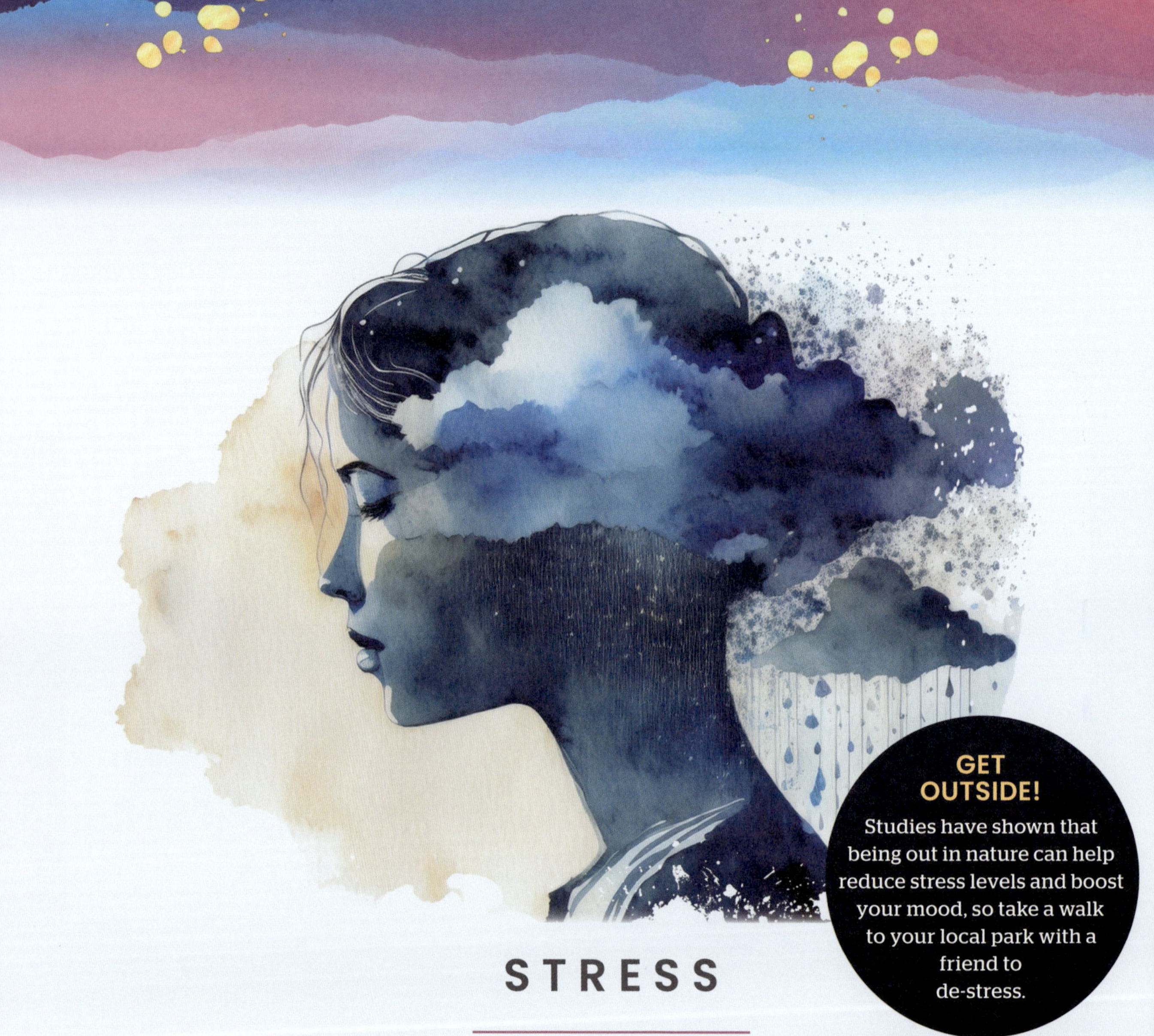

GET OUTSIDE!
Studies have shown that being out in nature can help reduce stress levels and boost your mood, so take a walk to your local park with a friend to de-stress.

STRESS

When you're under a lot of stress, it can trigger symptoms of anxiety. We all experience stress from time to time as a reaction to a particular incident, but if you're feeling stressed a lot of the time, or getting stressed more easily than usual, this is a sign that you need to take steps to manage your stress levels. Lifestyle interventions, like a healthy diet, exercise, and sleep, can help with resilience and calmness, whereas mindful movement and self-care can help to lessen the impact of stress when it happens.

It's important to identify the factors that contribute most to your stress, then you can think about what you can do to help reduce that trigger—can you delegate, for example, or do you need to break down a big task into smaller steps? Take some time to consider the biggest sources of stress in your life and what you can do about them. Use the opposite page to explore your thoughts.

Think about three things that make you feel stressed regularly.
Make a note of them below and then what you can do to lessen each stressor.

STRESSOR	STRESSOR	STRESSOR
....	....	....
....	....	....
What can I do to lessen this stress?	**What can I do to lessen this stress?**	**What can I do to lessen this stress?**
....	....	....
....	....	....
....	....	....
....	....	....

When you're stressed, how do you feel?
Make a note of both the physical and mental symptoms.

....

....

What could you do to feel calmer when you're under stress?

....

....

Social Support

UNDERSTAND THE IMPORTANCE OF HAVING A GOOD NETWORK AROUND YOU.

Social support refers to the role that friends, families, communities, and groups play when it comes to managing your anxiety. Having a good level of social support can enable you to have any practical help that you need, as well as reduce stress and improve coping mechanisms.

Sometimes the only people who understand how you're feeling and what you're going through are others in the same situation. Support groups can be a useful resource, enabling you to share your thoughts in a non-judgmental and compassionate environment. You can also share tips of what works for you and learn from others. These could be in-person groups in your local area, virtual groups held live at the same time each week, or online forums where you can discuss your thoughts whenever it suits you.

SUPPORT YOUR MENTAL HEALTH

Research shows that a lack of quality relationships, which help form social support systems, is associated with poorer mental health.

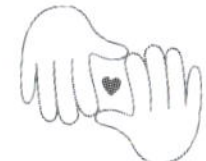

BUILD A SUPPORT SYSTEM

Take some time to think about who you could have in your support system. This usually includes any friends or family who you trust to understand your anxiety and know you can talk to without judgment. For some people, this may be enough, but it's also good to have a support system outside of your usual connections. For example, many people find they get a lot of support from clubs or communities they're part of. If you don't feel like you have anyone around you who can support you with your anxiety, see if there are any groups or activities in your area that can help.

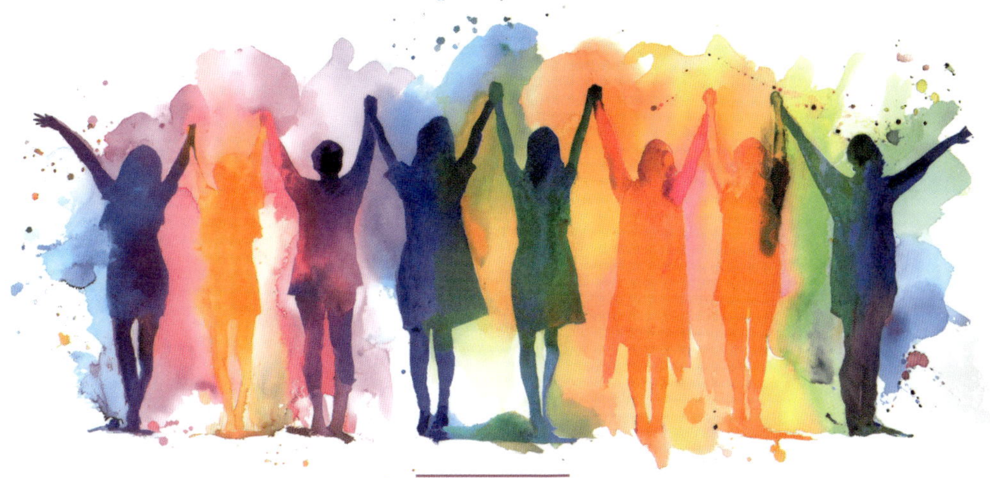

How do you feel about your current support system? Do you have enough support, or do you need to build your social network?

Make a list of people who are in your social support system. Write down the name of the person, group, or community, what type of support they offer, and how they help you.

ONE
Name
....
Type
(friend, group, club, etc.)
....
How they help me
....
....
....

TWO
Name
....
Type
(friend, group, club, etc.)
....
How they help me
....
....
....

THREE
Name
....
Type
(friend, group, club, etc.)
....
How they help me
....
....
....

FOUR
Name
....
Type
(friend, group, club, etc.)
....
How they help me
....
....
....

FIVE
Name
....
Type
(friend, group, club, etc.)
....
How they help me
....
....
....

SIX
Name
....
Type
(friend, group, club, etc.)
....
How they help me
....
....
....

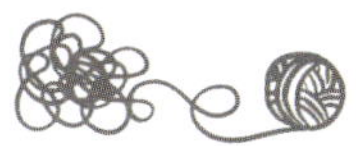

COMMUNICATE

Telling someone you have anxiety and explaining how it impacts your life can be a difficult task. Many people keep these thoughts to themselves or bottle up their feelings, but you need to be open and honest with your support network so they can help. Make sure you have the conversation in a private space at a time when you're both feeling calm and undistracted. Try to prepare before you speak to them to gather your thoughts. Are there specific triggers you've noticed? What areas of your life are you struggling with? How does your anxiety make you feel? Give them a chance to ask questions, so they can understand what you're dealing with and what you need from them. It can help to give specific examples of times when you've felt anxious, how that impacted you, and how they could have helped in that situation.

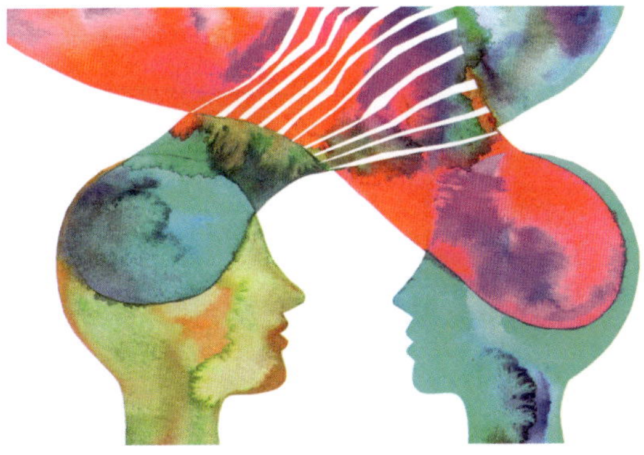

How does talking about your anxiety make you feel?

What sort of help would be beneficial from those in your support network? It might be that you need support with a specific task or just someone to listen when you're worried about something.

Build Mental Resilience

CREATE A POSITIVE MINDSET THAT HELPS YOU NAVIGATE LIFE'S CHALLENGES.

Resilience refers to your ability to face challenges, adapt to change, and bounce back. When you're feeling anxious, you might find your resilience is low, meaning it's harder to cope with obstacles, which can then increase your anxiety. Through self-care, self-awareness, acceptance, and gratitude, you can shift toward a more positive and resilient mindset.

EXPLORE SELF-COMPASSION

Feeling anxious can trigger a lot of negative self-talk. When something goes wrong, you might blame yourself for it happening or berate yourself for not coping with it better. When you're hard on yourself, it knocks your resilience and makes it more difficult to put situations into perspective. One of the first steps toward becoming more resilient is embracing self-compassion, which means to treat yourself with kindness and patience, rather than with negativity and guilt. It also means accepting your limitations and knowing when you need help, rather than trying to struggle through everything alone. These exercises can help you explore your relationship with yourself.

Imagine a friend is struggling with anxiety. What would you say to them? Would you treat them with kindness, compassion, and understanding?

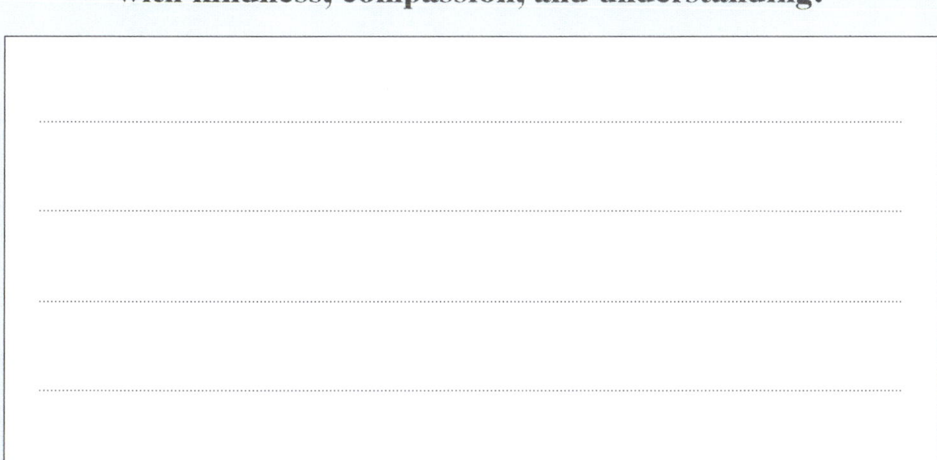

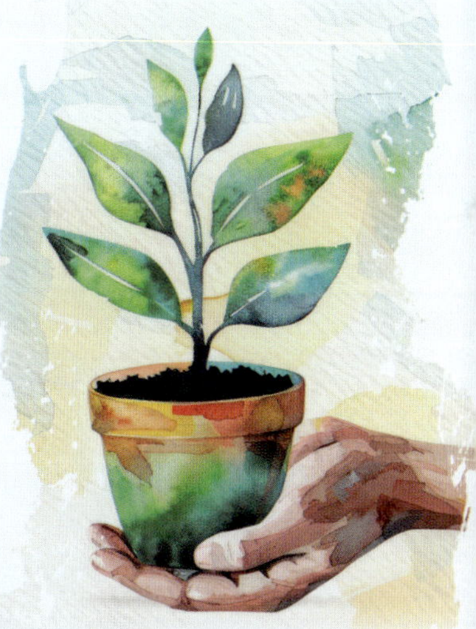

Now, apply that same kindness to yourself. Write down some negative thoughts you have noticed recently and think about how you can be kinder to yourself by replacing those thoughts with more compassionate ones. For example, "I messed up; I'm so stupid" could become "I made a mistake, but I tried my best."

Negative thought

Compassionate thought

Negative thought

Compassionate thought

Negative thought

Compassionate thought

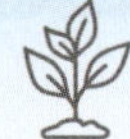

DEVELOP A GROWTH MINDSET

Our thoughts are powerful; they influence our emotions and actions. Our mindset is our way of thinking, determined by our beliefs and the way we perceive the world. A negative mindset focuses on unhelpful thoughts and only seeing the downside. A positive mindset is the opposite, thinking more optimistically, looking for solutions rather than problems. When it comes to building resilience, we want to foster a growth mindset, not a fixed mindset. A fixed mindset is when we believe we can't change anything, whether that's our beliefs, abilities, or skills. This leads to negative self-talk, as well as making it harder to adapt to change. A growth mindset, however, is when we believe change is possible—failure is an opportunity to learn, critical feedback can help you improve, and you can always develop skills and abilities. Building a growth mindset makes you more adaptable and resilient. Try these exercises to cultivate a more positive mindset.

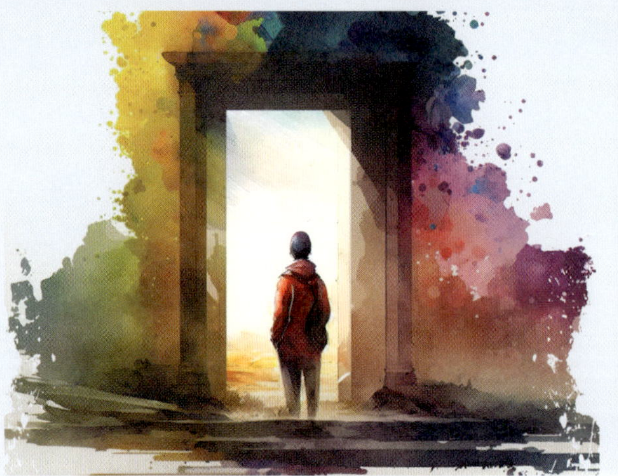

Write down a fixed belief you have about yourself; for example, "I'm not good enough to get a promotion at work."

How can you overturn this fixed belief?
Think about any positive attributes, feedback you've had, and examples that challenge the belief you've identified. For example, "I work hard, my colleagues say I'm a team player, and I'm willing to learn new skills."

Now rewrite your fixed belief into a growth belief—for example, "I know if I work hard and develop my skills, I will be ready to go forward for a promotion."

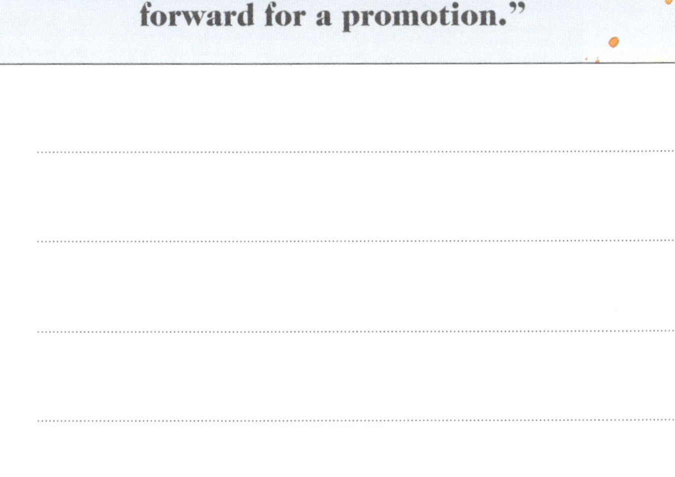

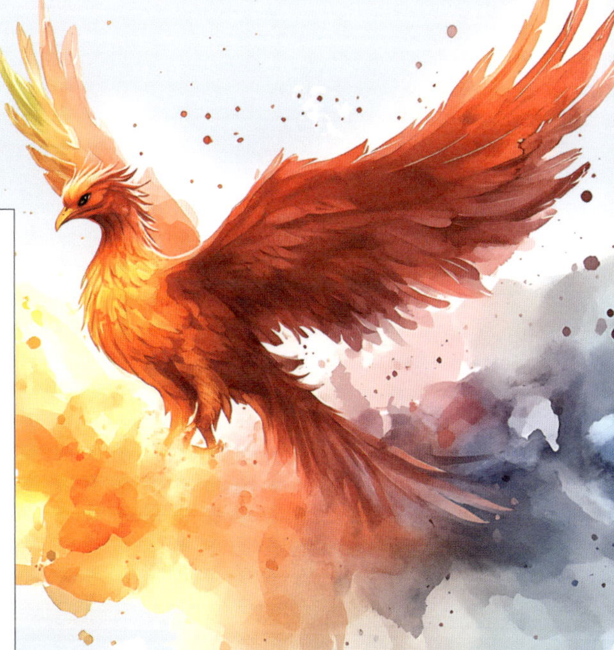

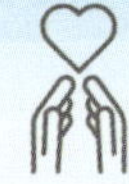

PRACTICE GRATITUDE

When you're anxious, you might focus a lot on the negative, and this can make you forget about the good in your life. Practicing gratitude can help you become more resilient by reminding you that even when things are hard, there is still a lot to be thankful for. Being grateful for the little things in life can encourage you to feel more positive, improve your well-being, and make you feel generally happier.

Regular gratitude practice can help to combat a steady stream of negative thinking, breaking those patterns and grounding you in the moment. When you're not used to practicing gratitude, it can feel a little forced and you might struggle to recognize and appreciate the positive. It's not about being relentlessly positive or minimizing difficult experiences, but gratitude can give you both perspective and hope, moving your focus away from your anxiety and toward gentle appreciation.

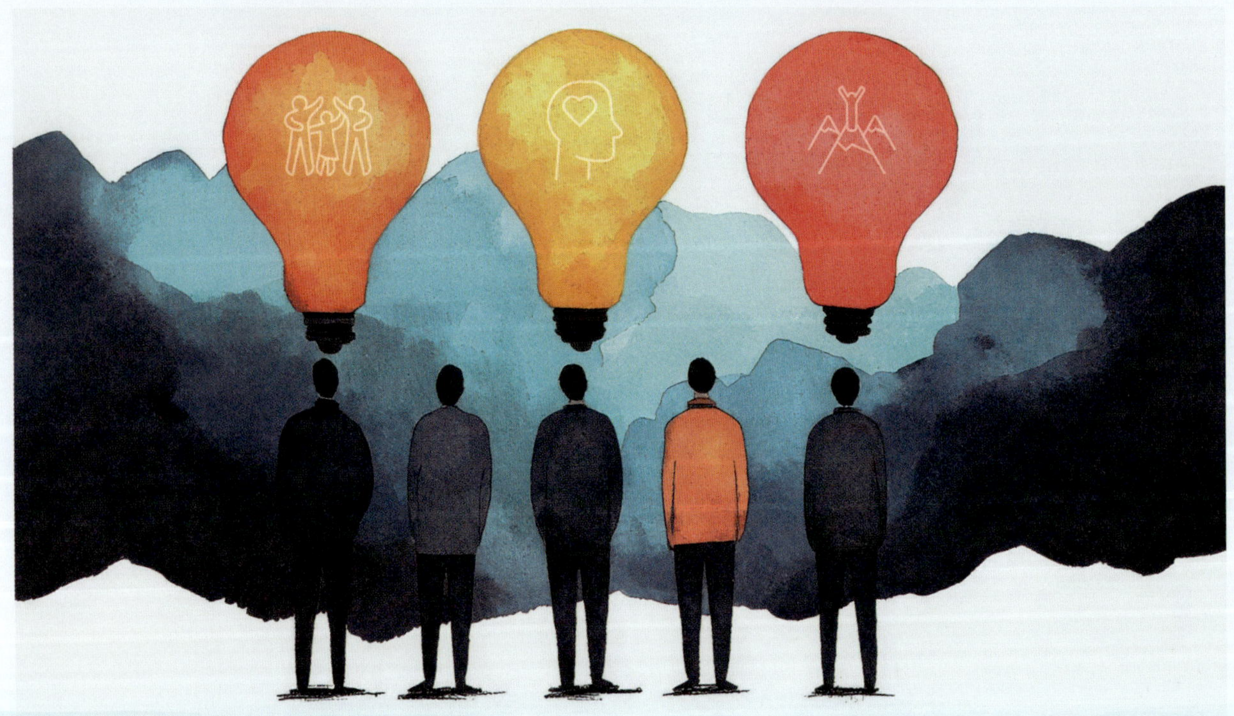

Think of something that has made you anxious or worried recently. Try to write down anything about that experience you could be grateful for. For example, did you learn something from the experience?

Make a gratitude list. Write down anything in your life that you're grateful for, no matter how big or small. Refer back to this on the days when you find it difficult to practice gratitude.

I am grateful for...

I am grateful for...

I am grateful for...

I am grateful for...

I am grateful for...

I am grateful for...

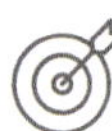

SETTING GOALS

Having small goals can help you focus, increase motivation, and build confidence.

When you feel anxious, tasks and goals can suddenly seem overwhelming, which can make it hard to get started on anything. Learning to take a large task and break it down into smaller steps can help to give you purpose and direction, motivating you to take that first push forward, and easing your symptoms. Rather than worrying that you'll never reach your goal, you focus on only thinking about the next step. Over time, you will become more confident in taking each step, and you may find that completing each task helps to give you extra resilience too. Here we give you space to identify some key goals and break them down into smaller, more manageable steps.

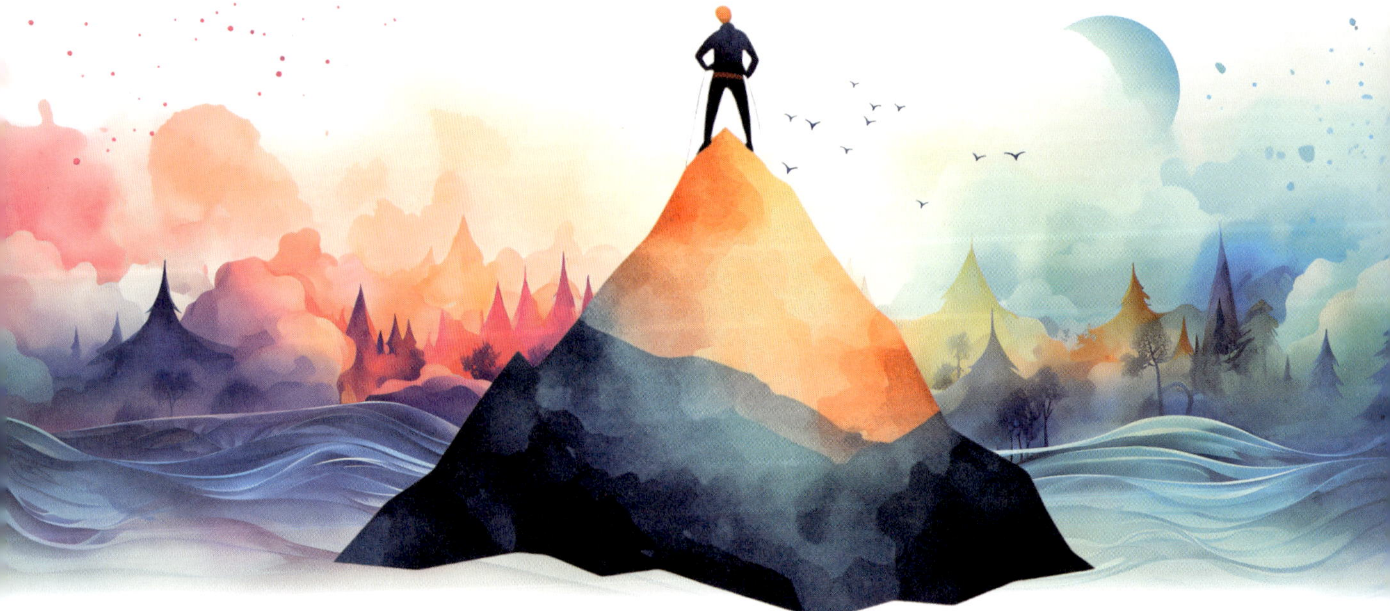

"Rather than worrying that you'll never reach your goal, you only think about the next step"

Write down some big goals or tasks, and then think about how you can break them down into smaller, more manageable steps.

BIG GOAL

Steps to reach my goal

BIG GOAL

Steps to reach my goal

BIG GOAL

Steps to reach my goal

LEARN AS YOU GO

When you achieve a step, use it as a learning experience, reflecting on what you've achieved and how it made you feel. Celebrate your successes, as no matter how small the step you've taken, you're going in the right direction, and that's ace!

Hobbies & Interests

TAKE THE TIME TO DO THINGS YOU ENJOY EVERY DAY TO MANAGE YOUR ANXIETY.

When you're feeling anxious, it can become harder to make time for yourself. But having a variety of hobbies and interests can help you to manage the condition. How much time do you currently put aside to take part in your hobbies and interests? The answer is usually "not enough," but hobbies can help to improve your mood, give you a sense of well-being, and boost your self-confidence. It might be that you don't have any particular hobbies or interests that you pursue at the moment, and the thought of trying something new feels overwhelming. However, trying a new hobby, especially if it's out of your comfort zone, can give you a goal to work toward and offer a sense of achievement when you do it. Take this time to think about what hobbies and interests you already have, as well as those that you'd like to try.

BE CREATIVE

Research shows that creative hobbies such as reading for pleasure, drawing, and listening to music can all help reduce symptoms of anxiety and improve your mood.

What hobbies and interests do you currently have (even if you don't always make time to do them)?

....

....

....

....

Disregarding all external factors (like time, budget or convenience), what hobbies or interests would you like to try? Put a check next to the ones that appeal, and add any others in the blank spaces.

- ☐ Learning a language
- ☐ Playing a musical instrument
- ☐ Gardening
- ☐ Sewing, knitting, or crocheting
- ☐ Painting
- ☐ Photography
- ☐ Cooking or baking
- ☐ Walking or hiking
- ☐ Taking up a new sport
- ☐ ....
- ☐ ....
- ☐ ....

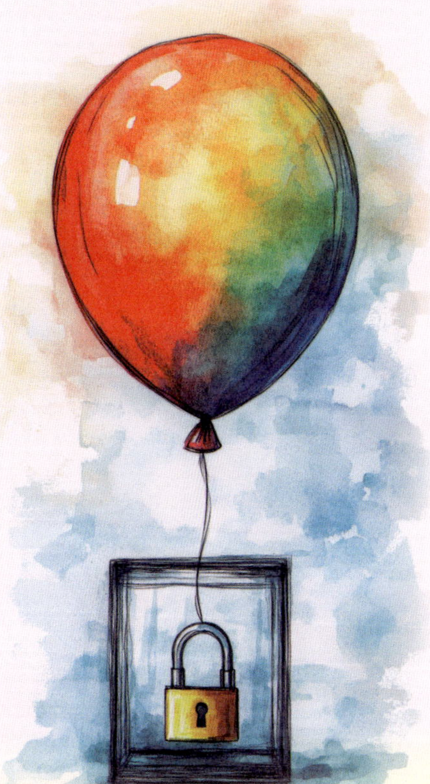

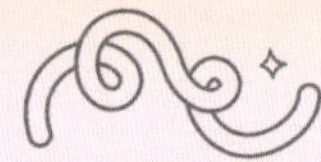

CHALLENGES AND OBSTACLES

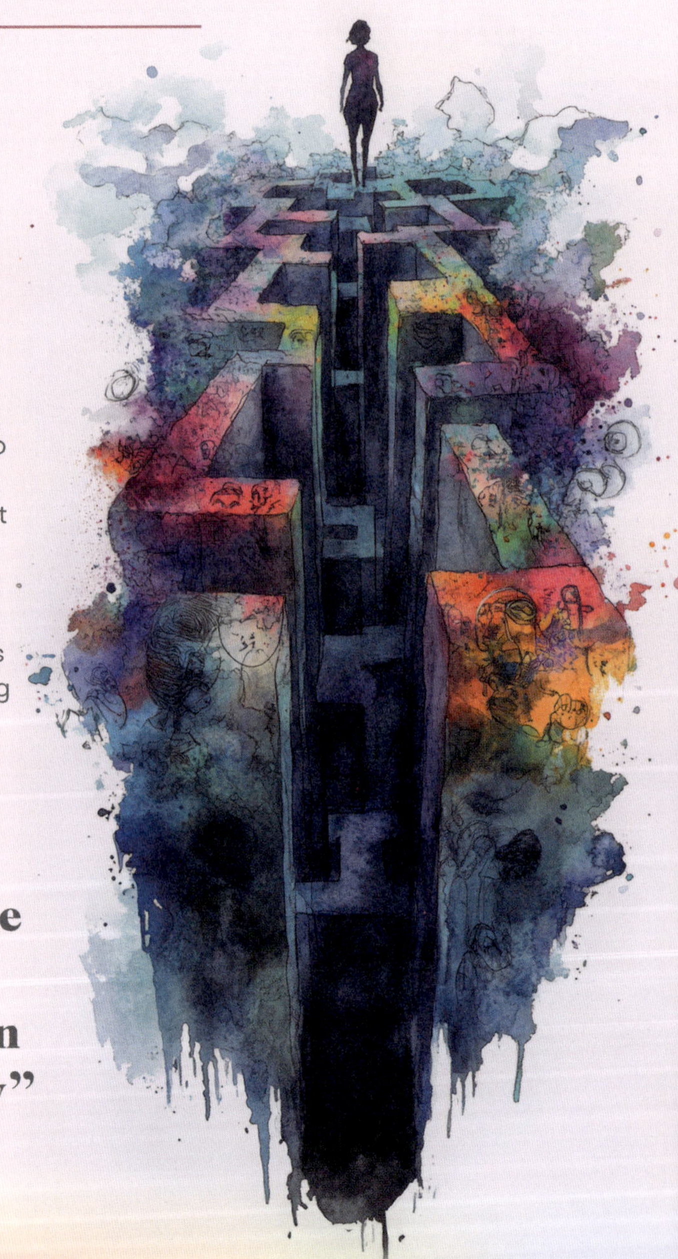

You've identified what interests you want to pursue, so now you need to think about the challenges that are preventing you from doing them. You may feel a sense of guilt for taking time to do something you enjoy, especially if you have work and caring responsibilities. Or maybe you have a fear of failure or being judged.

Many of us also feel anxious about interacting with a new hobby, especially if it means going to a club, group, or class with people you haven't met before. These obstacles can make it difficult to step outside your comfort zone, but it can also be hard to engage with existing hobbies and interests, even when it's something you enjoy. Think about the obstacles and challenges you're facing that are preventing you from doing existing or new hobbies, then come up with a plan for how you can break these down into smaller steps to make everything feel less overwhelming.

"It can be hard to engage with existing hobbies and interests, even when it's something you enjoy"

What obstacles and challenges do you currently face when it comes to engaging in hobbies and interests? This could be things like a lack of time, not prioritizing interests, social anxiety, or not knowing how to get started.

Focusing on your biggest obstacle, see if you can break it down into actionable steps that you can tackle one by one. For example, if you want to take a class to learn a new hobby but you feel overwhelmed, could you find an instruction video to practice at home first, or ask a friend to go with you?

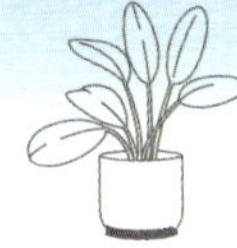

CREATE A CALM HOME

Create a stress-free sanctuary with these anxiety-busting décor tips.

Up your greenery game
Indoor plants not only provide an instant visual pick-me-up, but they also help us feel calmer and more relaxed in the long term. Decorating your shelves and sideboards with varieties that thrive inside can therefore create a soothing environment in which to unwind and relax.

Load up on lavender
Also known as nature's miracle plant, lavender has been proven to relieve symptoms of anxiety and lower stress. Take note and pepper your drawers with the herb, light lavender-scented candles, or simply decorate your space with fresh or dried cuts of the pretty purple blooms.

Decorate with blue
Colors have a powerful impact on our mood. So if you're curating a restful retreat, you should opt for a soft, neutral palette over loud, eye-popping hues like red and orange. Blue in particular has been proven to reduce blood pressure, lower stress, and promote feelings of sleepiness.

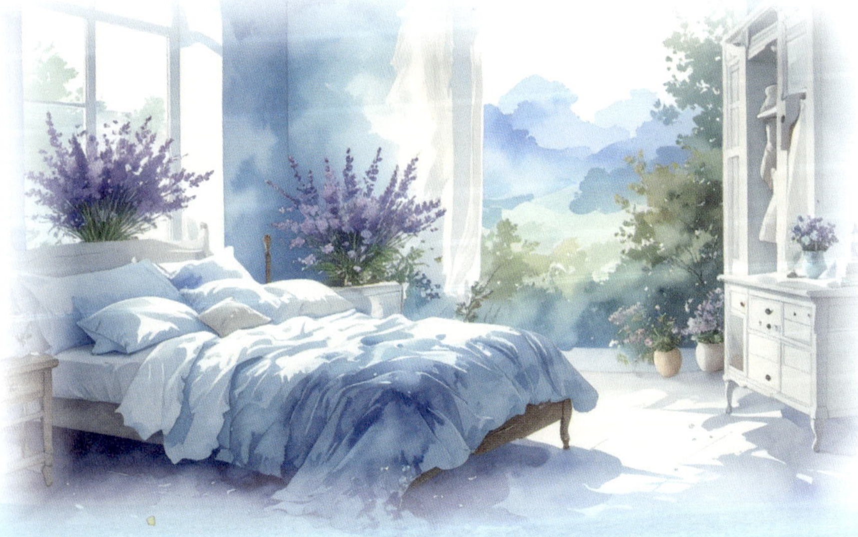

Limit use of patterns
Our senses can be sent into overdrive by an excessive use of polka dots, stripes, and paisley print. To create a calm and balanced space, it pays to banish any busy embellishments and flamboyant flourishes in favor of plain blocks of color and simple detailing.

Pile on soft textiles
People with anxiety have an

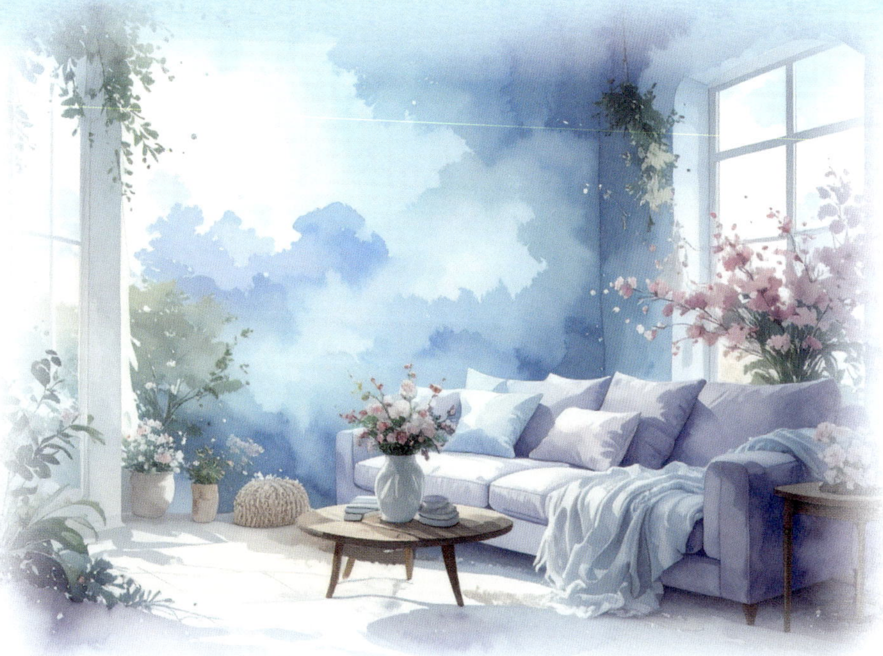

increased sensitivity and appreciation of soft fabrics. Take this as a design directive to add some soothing textiles to your home. Think faux fur cushions, plush fleecy throws, sumptuous rugs, and weighted blankets to make your space cozy.

Let in natural light
Not getting enough sunlight can lead to a vitamin D deficiency and a disturbed circadian rhythm, both of which have been linked to anxiety and depression. Opening your curtains and letting the natural light flood inside is therefore a key component of creating a tranquil space.

Stow away all the clutter
A messy house can make us feel tense and overwhelmed. Studies even show that living in a cluttered environment can increase the stress hormone cortisol. One fix is to invest in some smart storage solutions, while regular purges and opting for a less-is-more approach will never go amiss.

Buy some fresh flowers
Beautiful bouquets never fail to lift the spirits, and it's not just because of their good looks. Flowers release chemicals that signal the brain to release the feel-good hormone serotonin. So filling your space with freshly cut buds can actually have a positive impact on your mental well-being.

Cover up technology
Too much screen time has been linked to an increased risk of depression and anxiety, but a few small changes in the home can help limit your smart device usage. For example, make your bedroom a phone-free zone, store your laptop away, or hide your television behind a decorative screen.

Get a good bed
One of the best ways to help keep anxiety symptoms at bay is getting enough sleep. A comfortable mattress therefore can be considered the bedrock of a stress-free home. Be sure to pair yours with some soft and comforting bed linen for the ultimate night's sleep.

"Studies show that living in a cluttered environment can increase the stress hormone cortisol"

Try Another Way

ALTERNATIVE THERAPIES CAN HELP WITH ANXIETY. HERE ARE SOME THAT YOU CAN DO, LEARN, AND BUY YOURSELF.

Feeling anxious but don't want to wait for an appointment with the doctor or counselor? Why not go for some alternative remedies? These are treatments and practices known for their healing effects, but which fall outside of conventional medicine. So that could be mindfulness, meditation, visualization, massage, and acupuncture, to name a few. You can also use music and art, essential oils, herbs and crystals. These and many other therapies, practices, and products can help you with stress, negative thoughts, worry, and other difficult emotions that can cause anxiety. Some alternative therapies are based on mainstream science. Others on belief, tradition, mysticism, and some on fringe science—science that isn't accepted as science by mainstream scientists. Alternative therapies can help you relax, feel positive, clear your mind, and focus away from your problems. So if this sounds like it would be useful for you, let's take a look at what options there are.

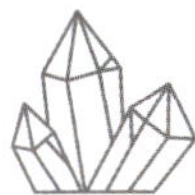

HEALING CRYSTALS

Crystals are minerals with atoms formed in a highly ordered, repeating pattern. These rocks are believed to possess helpful properties and have been used for therapeutic purposes for centuries.

The argument goes that crystals have a fixed energy pattern and unique energy field, which is what gives them special properties. It's believed that crystals work by affecting whatever is nearby, bringing balance and harmony to your own energy fields. This, in turn, helps you to stay calm. When our energies are unbalanced, so it's said, we're more likely to experience feelings of anxiety.

None of this is based on modern mainstream science. But people who use crystals say they have energies that help with different areas of life. Watch out for fake crystals made from glass, plastic, or that have been synthetically produced, though. Real crystals have imperfections and are cool to touch. Fakes scratch easily.

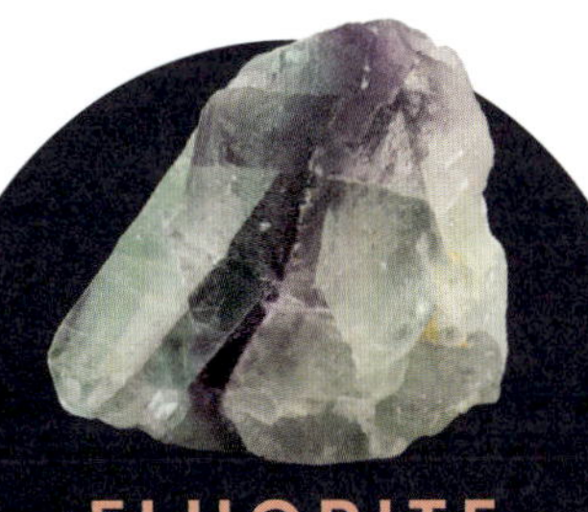

FLUORITE

Said to transform negative energy to positive. Will help you feel lighter and take life less seriously. Evokes a neutral state that can help you recognize your anxiety.

Tip Keep it next to your bed so it can work on your mind while you sleep.

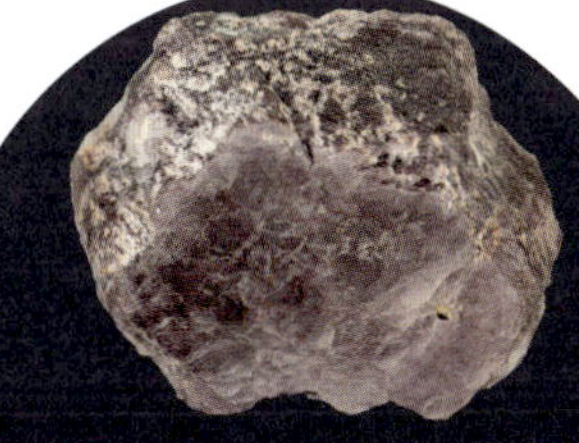

LEPIDOLITE

Contains lithium, a metallic element used in anti-anxiety medicine. Said to assist with breathing and release stress and worry by bringing you back to the present.

Tip Another one to keep by your bed for it to work while you sleep.

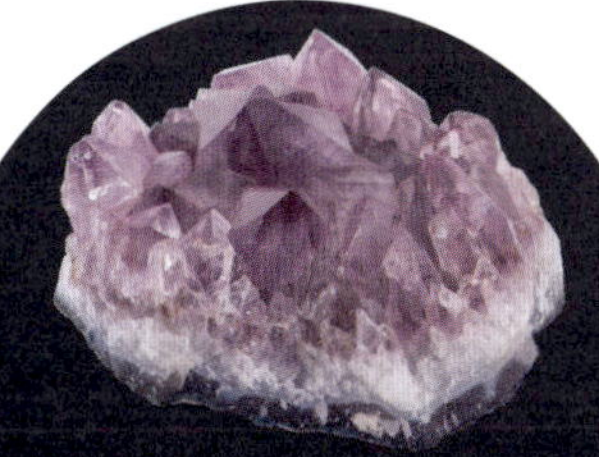

AMETHYST

Violet or purple quartz. Said to bring mental clarity, so can help you understand the source of your anxiety and promote peace of mind. The ancient Greeks believed it could keep you from getting drunk!

Tip Place it on your forehead to relax your mind. Hold it in your hand for clarity and focus.

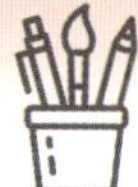

DRAW AWAY NEGATIVE THOUGHTS

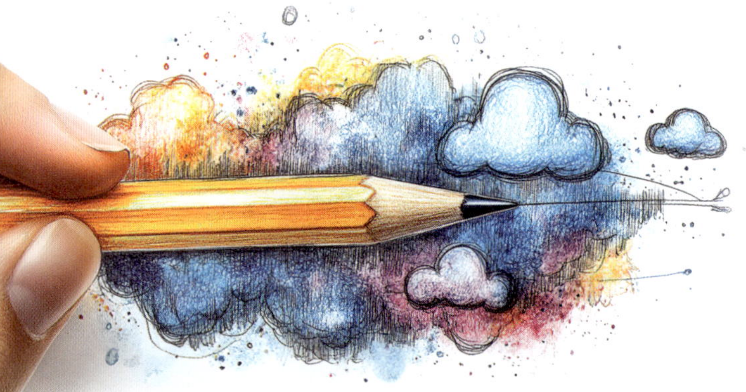

Ever wondered why you sometimes start drawing without realizing it when you feel a bit anxious? More likely a few scribbly doodles than a beautiful masterpiece.

It's because drawing is a great way of tuning into painful or difficult feelings. You can express how you feel without using words, get your mind away from uncontrollable anxious thoughts, and focus on something that you actually can control.

When drawing like this, negative thoughts might pop in your mind. When they do, either scribble down something that represents the thought and then move on to your next thought, or let the negative thought just float away. Immersed in your own world like this, distressing thoughts stop churning around in your head. You don't need to have something specific in mind to draw. Start off with a shape, a line, a scribble, or a color and don't worry about making mistakes. Just go with the flow of your mind and whatever needs to emerge, will emerge. And if you don't like to draw, you can always use clay, or cut images and shapes from magazines or colored paper to make a collage.

Use this space to draw something that calms you.

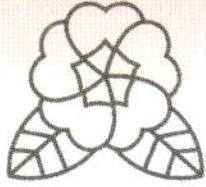

HERBAL BALANCE

People have been using herbs to treat illness for as long as there have been people. These herbs are called adaptogens and they interact with the processes within our bodies that balance hormones when we're stressed. The theory goes that adaptogens help us cope with challenging experiences better and for longer, as well as keeping our bodies balanced.

In many parts of the world herbs have always been an important part of medical care, particularly China and India. In the United States, herbs are growing in popularity and are available in stores and online. You can get them in capsules, teas, liquid drops, skin creams, as powder, or in dried plant extract.

Not all herbs are adaptogens. All adaptogens are nontoxic when taken in low doses.

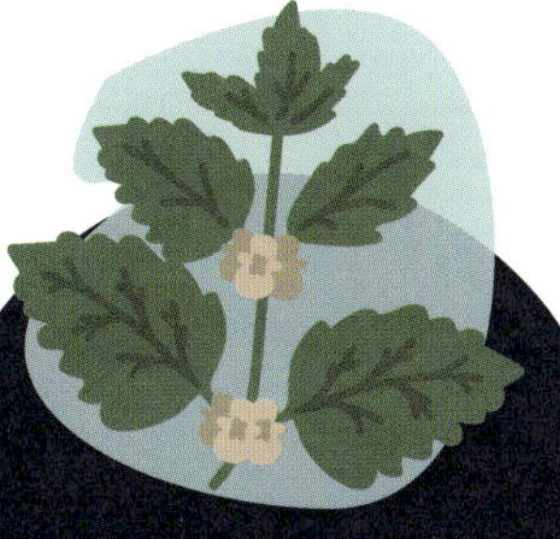

LEMON BALM

As part of the mint family, lemon balm is excellent for stomach complaints, but it also helps uplift your mood, works on the central nervous system to calm anxiety, and improves cognitive function.

Tip Add dried lemon balm to boiling water for a soothing sip, or find it in supplements and tea blends.

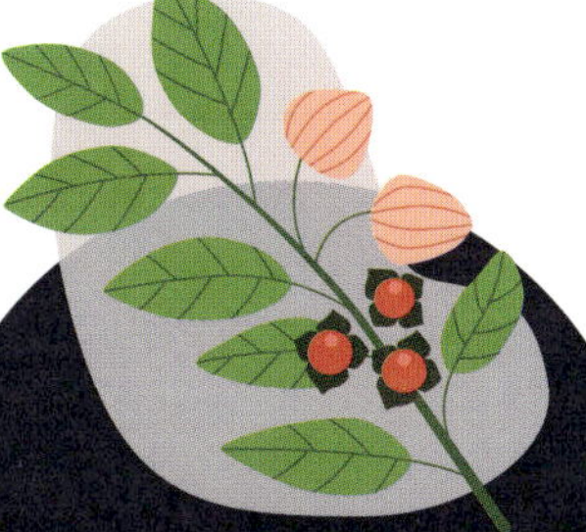

ASHWAGANDHA

This evergreen shrub has been used for over 5,000 years in India for its therapeutic value. It can reduce cortisol (stress hormone) levels in the blood, and reduce irritability and stress-related cravings.

Tip Add a cup of ashwagandha in powder form to a homemade smoothie, available in most health food stores.

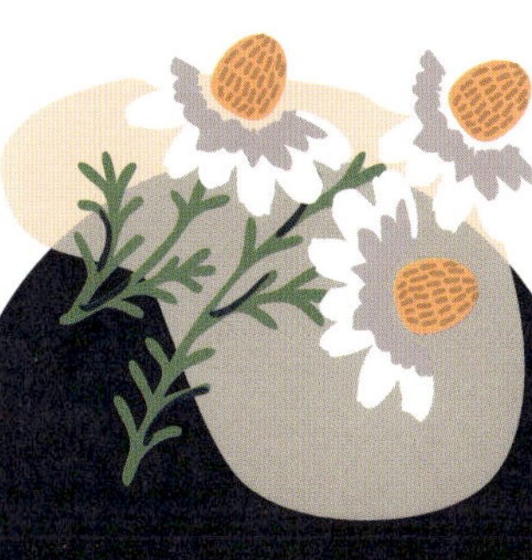

CHAMOMILE

Chamomile has been used since ancient times to treat nausea, stomach complaints, and help calm the mind and induce sleep.

Tip Dried chamomile can be added to boiling water to create a soothing tea. (Try a mix with lemon balm!)

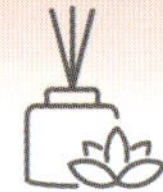

AROMATHERAPY—AN ANCIENT ART FOR ANXIETY

Aromatherapy is based on the therapeutic use of aromatic plants, a practice used since the beginning of human civilization.

According to many ancient texts, perfumes, oils, and ointments have been used in rituals, to cure diseases and to help people get what they want, whether that's money, health, or happiness.

You might have already used plant oils when you had a cold, in the form of a menthol-based ointment, but these powerful oils can aid the mind as much as the physical body. To reap the rewards of plant power, plant oils—which are called essential oils—can be inhaled or applied to the skin. You can buy handy devices such as electric diffusers, use a candle and burner, or simply add to hot water and breathe in, just like you do when you are sick. Essential oils can also be applied to clothing or rubbed into the skin (always mixing with a carrier oil like olive, jojoba, coconut oil, or a scentless balm such as petroleum jelly) but should never be swallowed.

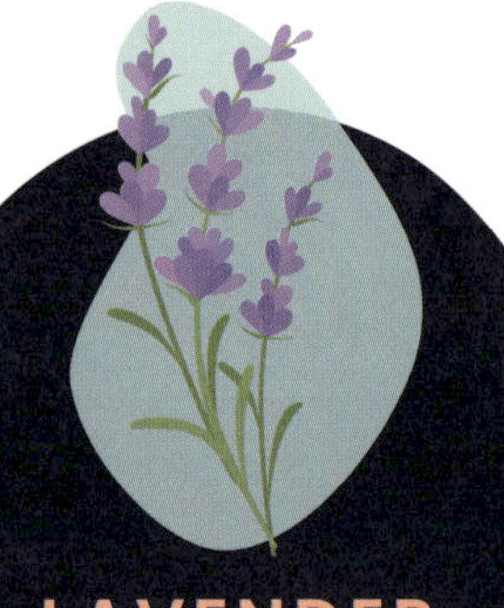

LAVENDER

Works on the brain to reduce the fight-or-flight stress response.

How to use Try diluted and applied to your pulse points, in a pillow spray or add essential oil to a warm bath.

Cautions Can cause nausea and should be used diluted on skin.

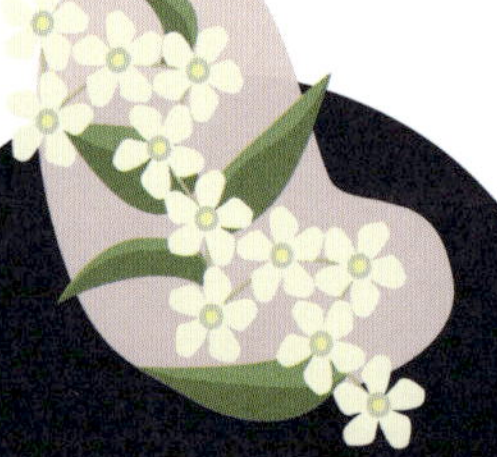

JASMINE

Calms the nervous system without causing sleepiness. Makes you feel more positive and energetic.

How to use Add to a plain carrier oil (such as grapeseed, jojoba, or almond) and massage into your skin.

Cautions Can cause allergic reactions on the skin—never apply directly!

SWEET ORANGE

Soothes nervous system, reduces pulse rate, and promotes healthy lymphatic flow.

How to use Use in a diffuser or add to a warm bath to boost your mood!

Cautions Can cause burns on the skin when exposed to sunlight, so use SPF if you add to your bath. Can irritate nose and throat if inhaled or swallowed. Apply diluted.

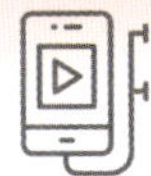

TAKE IN A FEW SOUNDS

Upbeat music makes you feel optimistic and positive, we know that, right? But did you know that slower-tempo music can help soothe or release stress?

Not that really mournful stuff where everyone is lamenting about how terrible life and the world is, around some slow melody. Forget all that stuff. Instead try Native American, Celtic, flute, ambient, light jazz, classical—even sounds of running water, rain, and storms, or nature. There are so many different types of music for you to choose from, so try a few out and discover the particular style that feels right for you. Instrumentals are more useful than the songs with lyrics or repetitive, catchy rhythms and melodies.

Listening to music helps with anxiety because it can lower your heart rate, reduce cortisol levels (the chemical we produce when we're stressed), and release endorphins (chemicals in the brain) that improve our sense of well-being. It can also help you fall asleep easier.

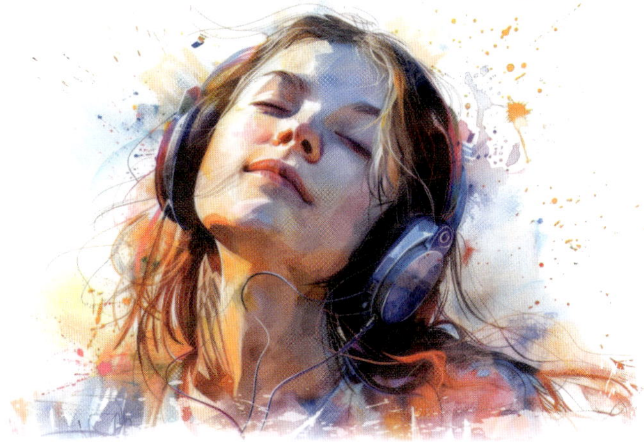

Make a list of five songs that make you feel at peace.

1. ....

2. ....

3. ....

4. ....

5. ....

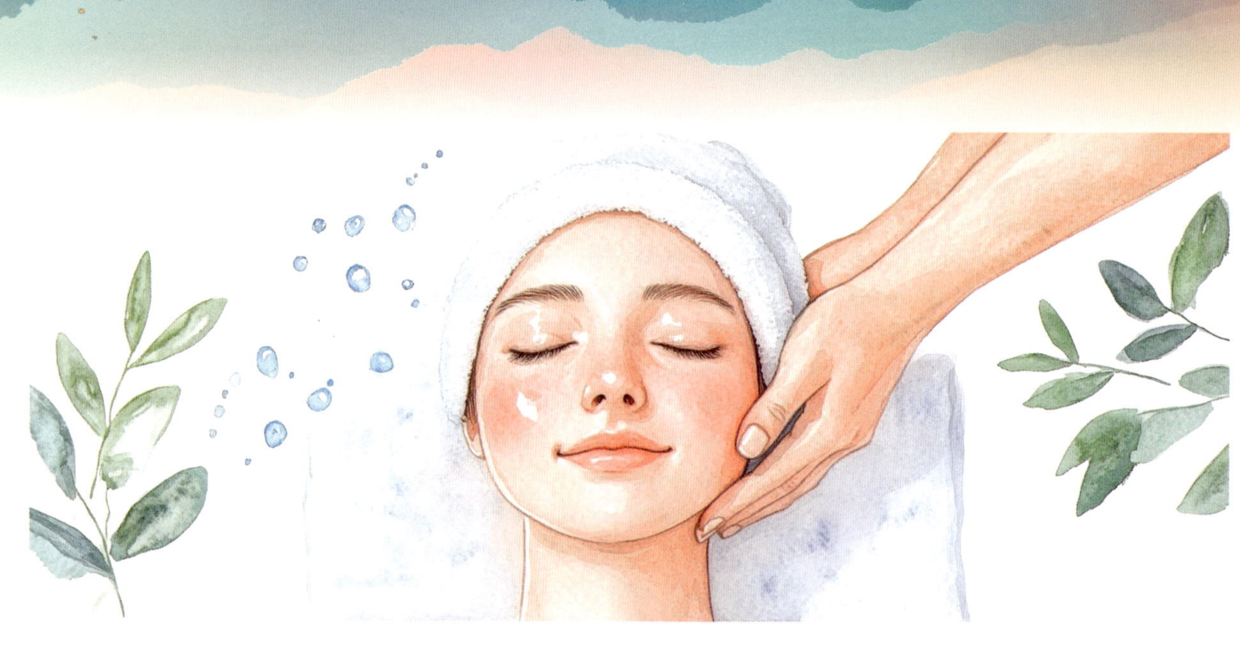

RELEASE THE PRESSURE

Physical touch is healing. It calms our central nervous system and slows our heartbeat. This could be a simple hug from a friend, a gentle hand squeeze from a family member, or a more elaborate form of touch healing, such as massage, reflexology, or acupuncture.

Massage stimulates parts of the brain that regulate emotions and stress response. It also reduces levels of the stress hormone cortisol, and stimulates our parasympathetic nervous system to keep us in the rest and digest state, rather than fight or flight.

Reflexology is a system of massage based on the theory that there are reflex points on the feet, hands, and head linked to every part of the body. The foot contains up to 7,000 nerves, each one corresponding to a different gland organ or muscle in the body. If the body is out of balance, problems can occur.

Acupuncture is an ancient practice where needles are inserted into pressure points on the body. In traditional Chinese medicine, these points stimulate blocked or interrupted qi (vital life energy) and promote healing. In the West, acupuncture is believed to stimulate the nervous system.

For all of these treatments you'd need a qualified therapist. But you can feel some benefit if you stimulate the pressure points yourself.

There's a point between your eyebrows, another in the upper shell of your ear, in the hollow part on the inner lobe, and two more on each foot just below the join of your big toe and second toe, above the bone in the hollow part. All these are said to help with anxiety.

To stimulate these points, run your finger along the area of your body until you find the point.

On the feet, apply firm, deep pressure to the point, either using your thumb, finger, or knuckle. Keep this pressure applied for four to five seconds.

With the ear point, apply firm, gentle pressure in a circular motion for two minutes. Do the same for the eyebrow point, but for five to ten minutes.

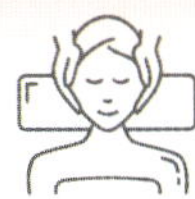

FACIAL MASSAGE TECHNIQUES FOR ANXIETY

You can gain a lot of calm from a simple facial massage. Repeat all of these for some stress and tension relief, to center your mind, and lessen headaches and neck pains.

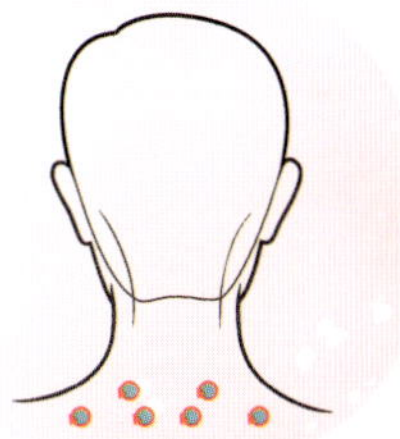

NECK AND SHOULDERS

An overall reliever; reach back to massage the base of your neck and shoulders in circular motions. Tip: some oil or moisturizer may make this more comfortable.

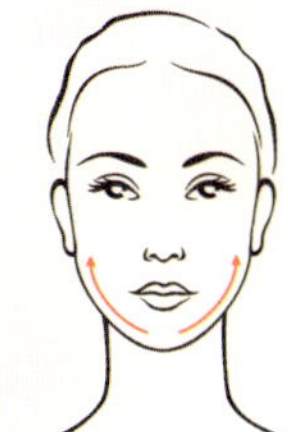

JAW RELEASE

Starting from the chin, push both hands upward along your jawline to your ear, then bring them down the sides of your neck. Use the most comfortable pressure.

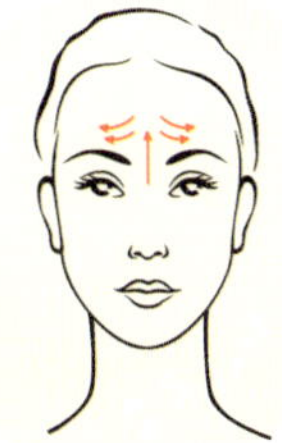

BROW SQUEEZE

This is a nice little stress reliever—start at the bridge of your nose and gently press your eyebrows between thumb and forefinger, working toward the ears.

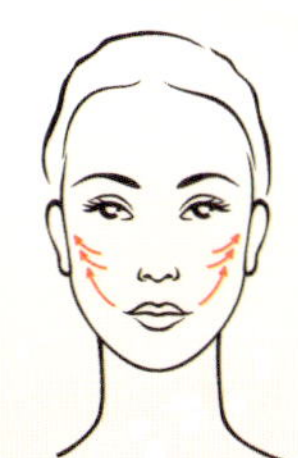

TAPPING

Tapping has been clinically proven to lower stress hormones. Using the tips of your fingers, start at your cheek bones and gently tap outward to your ears.

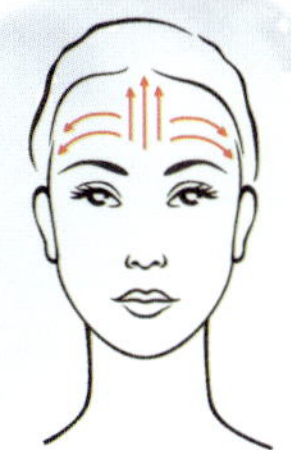

FOREHEAD SWEEP

Using the tips of your fingers, start applying pressure at the bridge of your nose and gently run upward, over your forehead and into your hairline, one hand after the other.

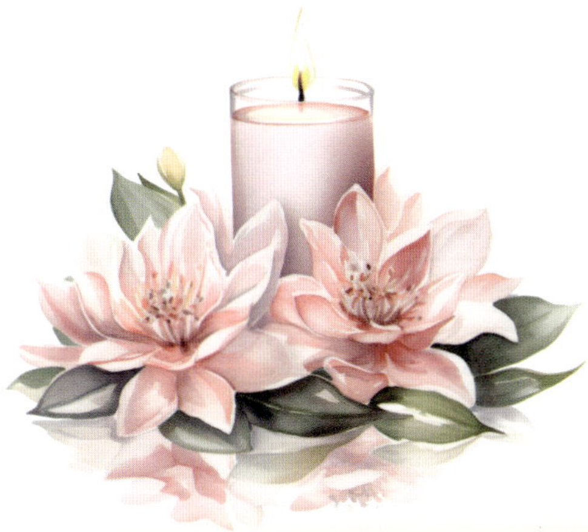

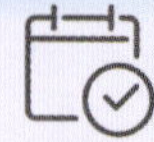

TRACK YOUR ANXIETY

Keep a log of your sleep, nutrition, exercise, anxiety, and time spent on yourself for a week to determine which areas you need to focus on.

WEEK BEGINNING 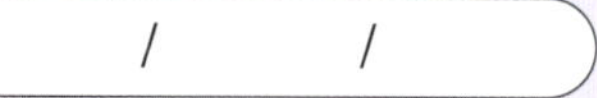

This week's anxiety triggers

◇ ....

◇ ....

◇ ....

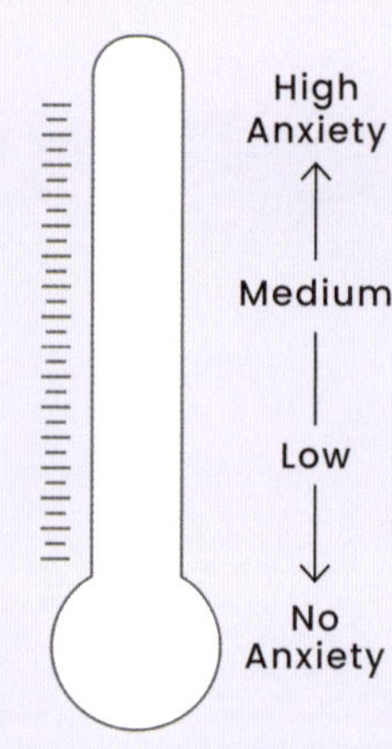

Sleep tracker

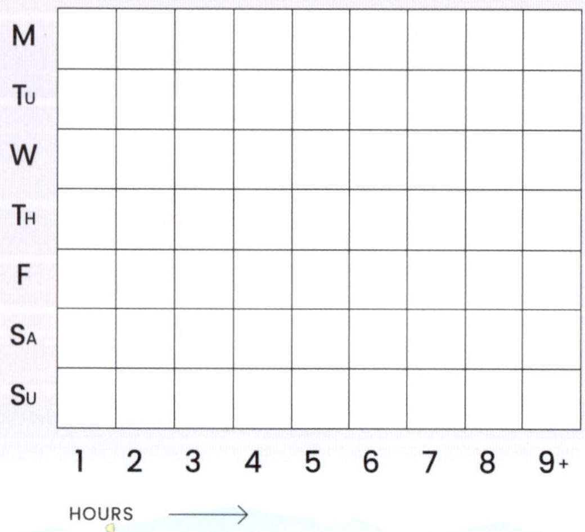

Diet & nutrition tracker

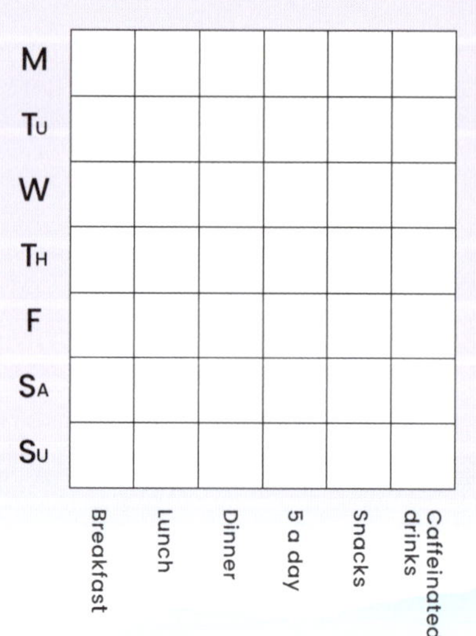

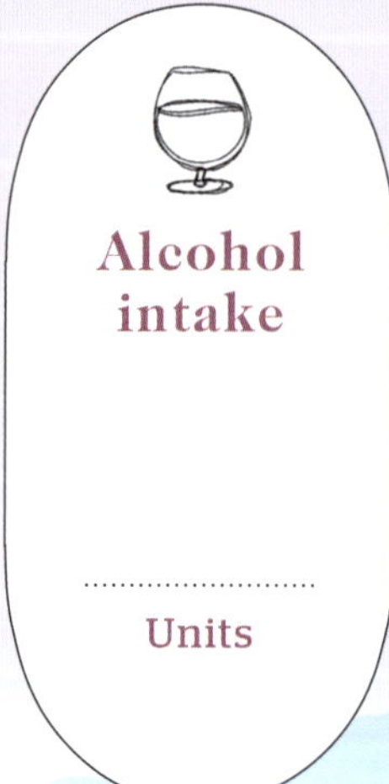

Water intake

GLASSES →

M	Tu	W	Th	F	Sa	Su
1	1	1	1	1	1	1
2	2	2	2	2	2	2
3	3	3	3	3	3	3
4	4	4	4	4	4	4
5	5	5	5	5	5	5
6	6	6	6	6	6	6
7	7	7	7	7	7	7
8	8	8	8	8	8	8

Social activity

Who did you see and what did you do?	How did it make you feel?

I am grateful for...

Exercise tracker

	Exercise	Feeling before	Feeling afterward
M			
Tu			
W			
Th			
F			
Sa			
Su			

Hobbies

Activity	How did it make you feel?

Reflect

How have you tried to manage your anxiety this week, what was the outcome, and what have you learned?

Art to reduce anxiety

Art will not only help you to slow down and take a breath, but it can help ease your anxiety. Color in these pages to calm yourself down and lift your mood.

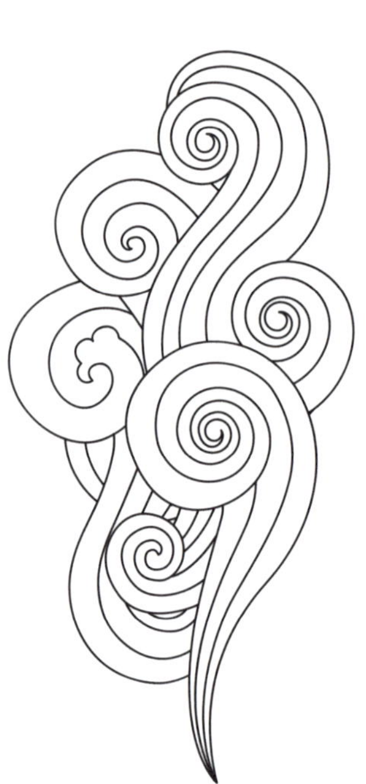

Panic attacks produce hyperventilation. Hyperventilation floods our muscles with oxygen, making us ready to fight or run away. But in a panic attack, there is nothing to run away from. Our deep brain is preparing us for a situation from our deep past, when what we are actually facing is the fear of giving a presentation or nerves before an exam, for example. The situations that produce anxiety in the modern world are rarely resolved by fighting or running away.

One way to tell our amygdala that there really is nothing to worry about is to control our breath. By controlling our breathing we can nudge the brain and nervous system out of the flight/fight response. To do so, we need to change the breath pattern into an in-breath to a slow count of four, and an out-breath to a slow count of four, preferably through the nose. It's important that the count is the same length for both.

This slow, even breathing will send a message through the body to the deep brain: there is no emergency, switch off the danger hormones.

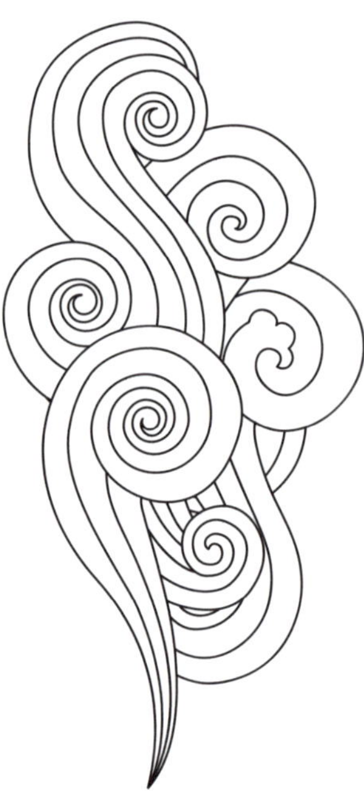

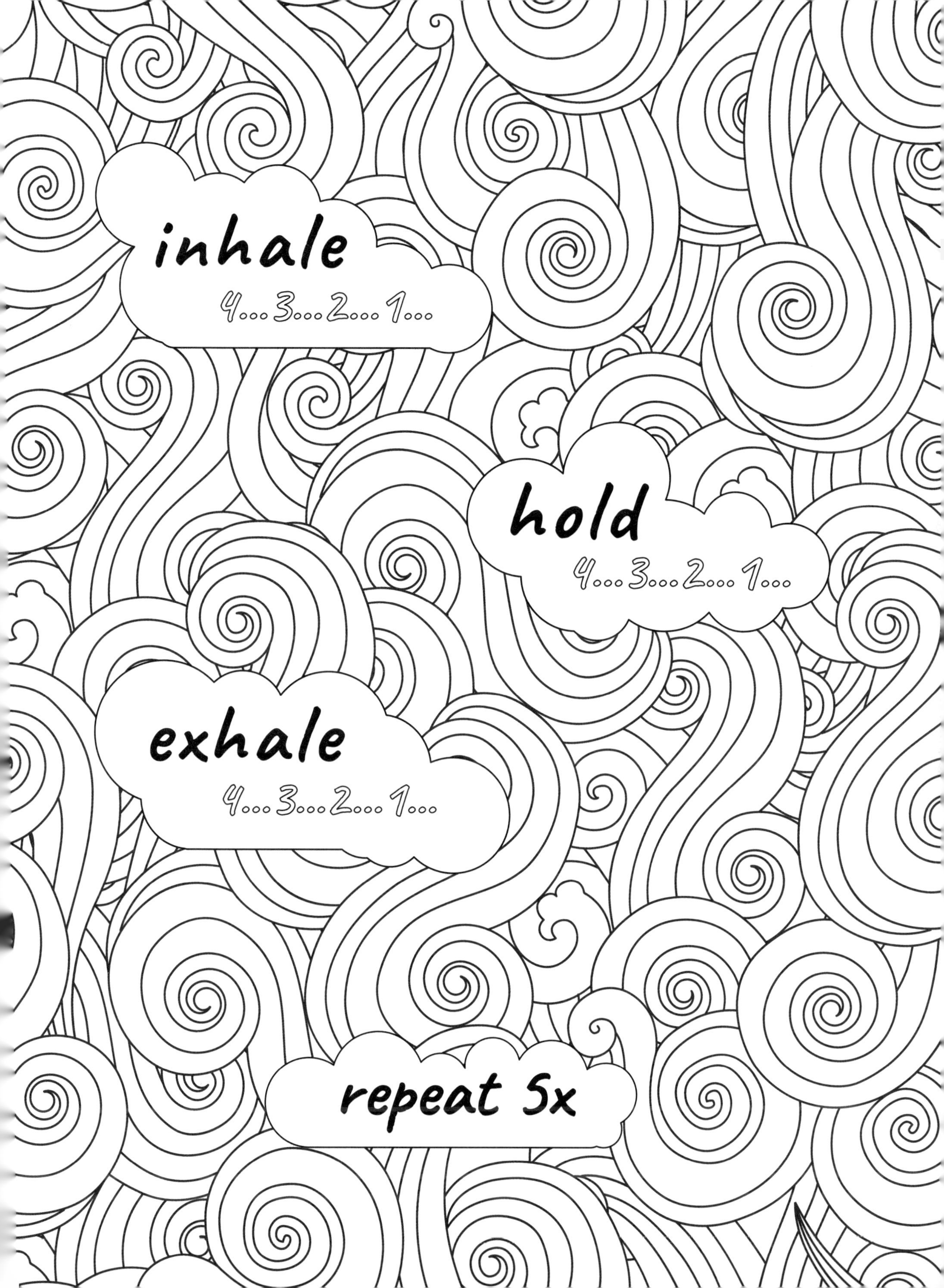
inhale
4... 3... 2... 1...
hold
4... 3... 2... 1...
exhale
4... 3... 2... 1...
repeat 5x

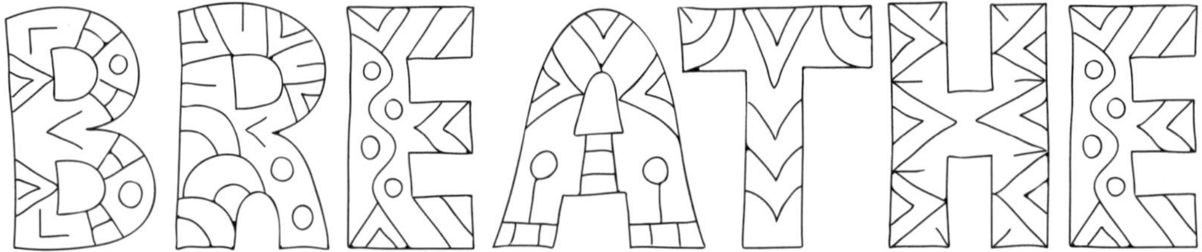
BREATHE

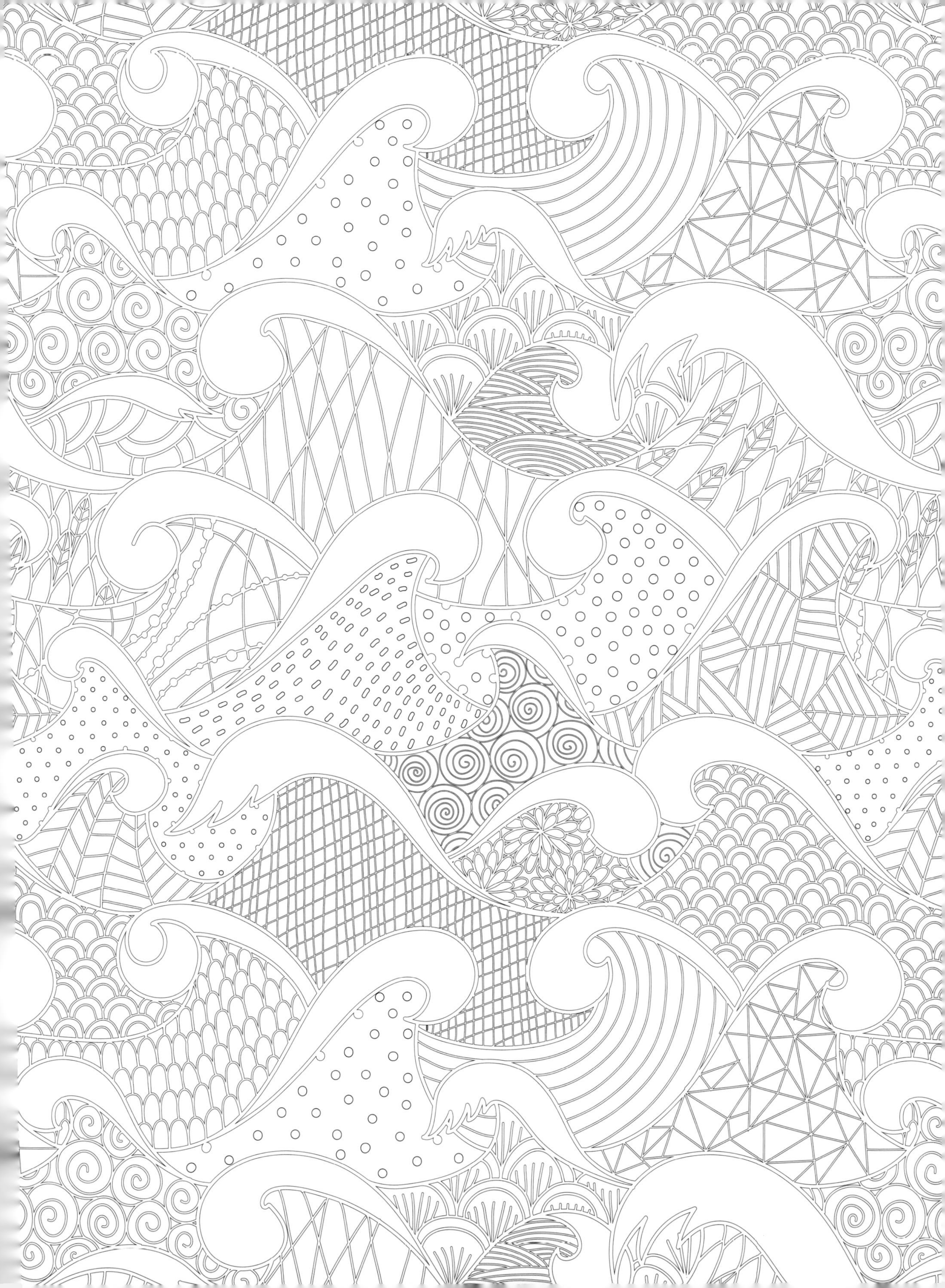

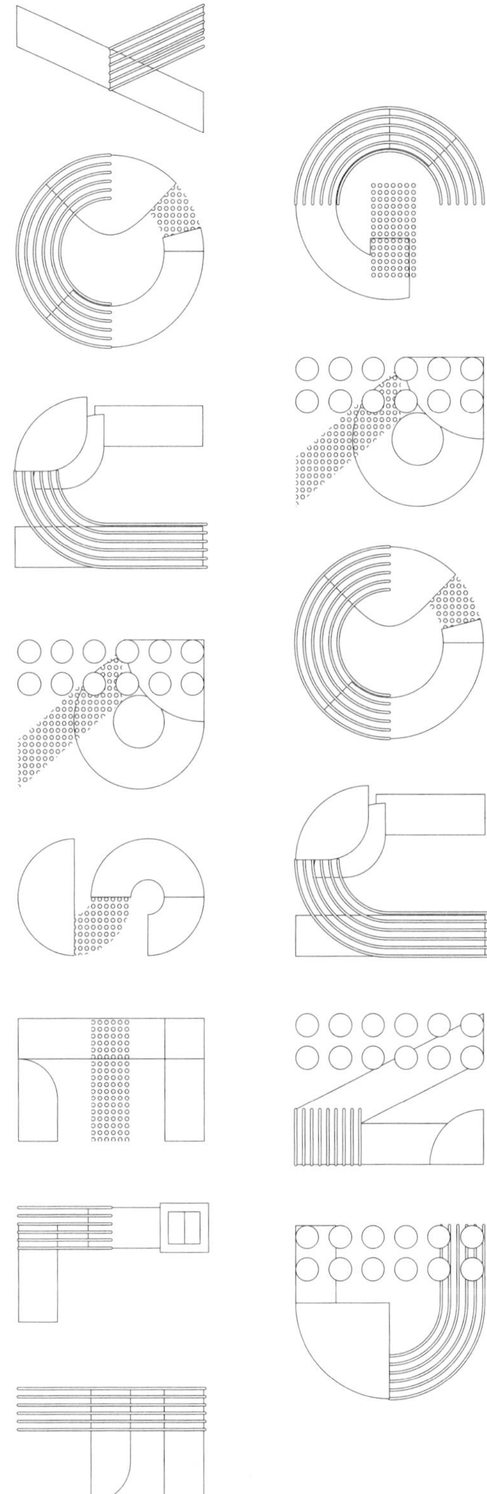

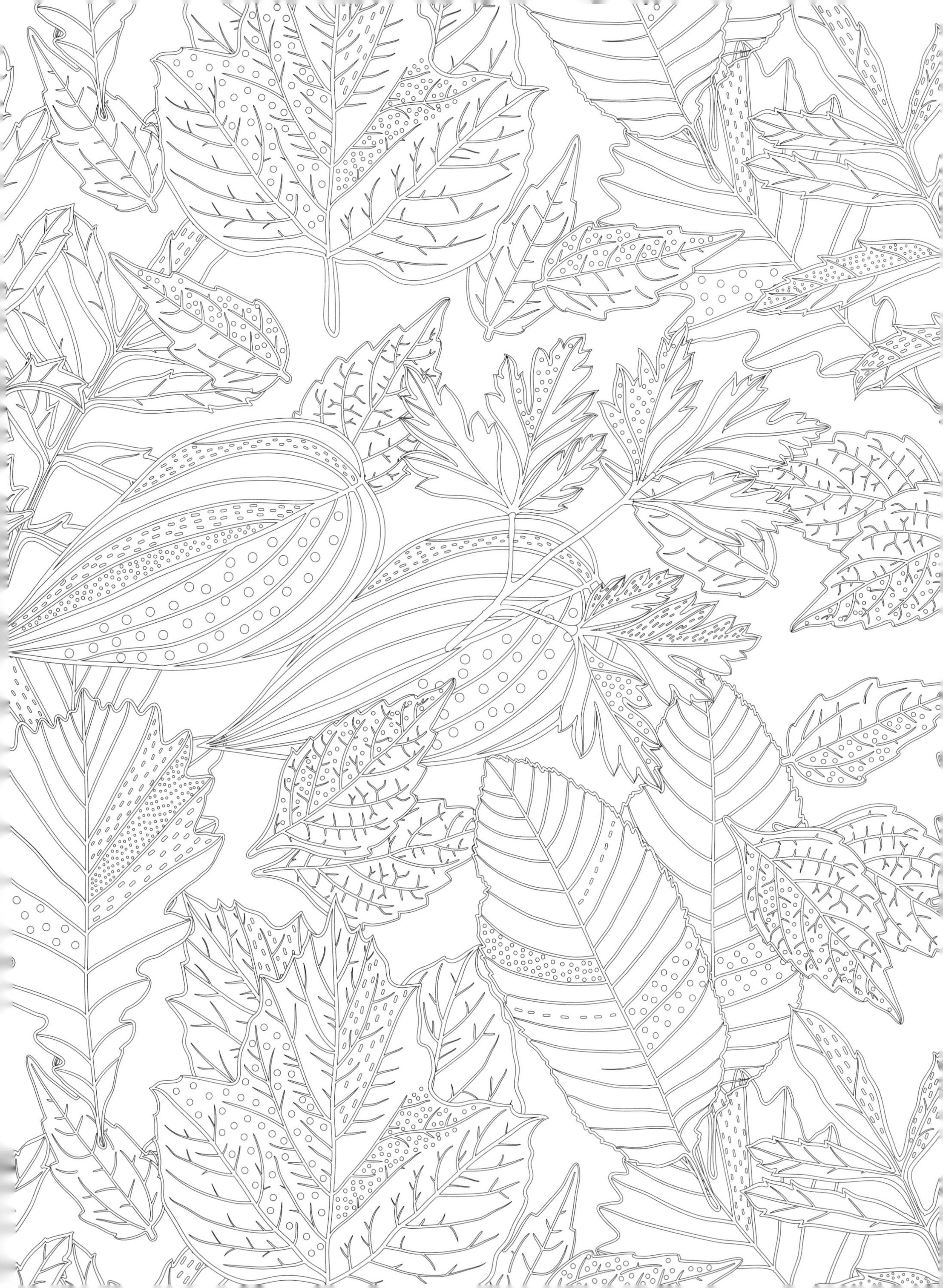

FIND
PEACE

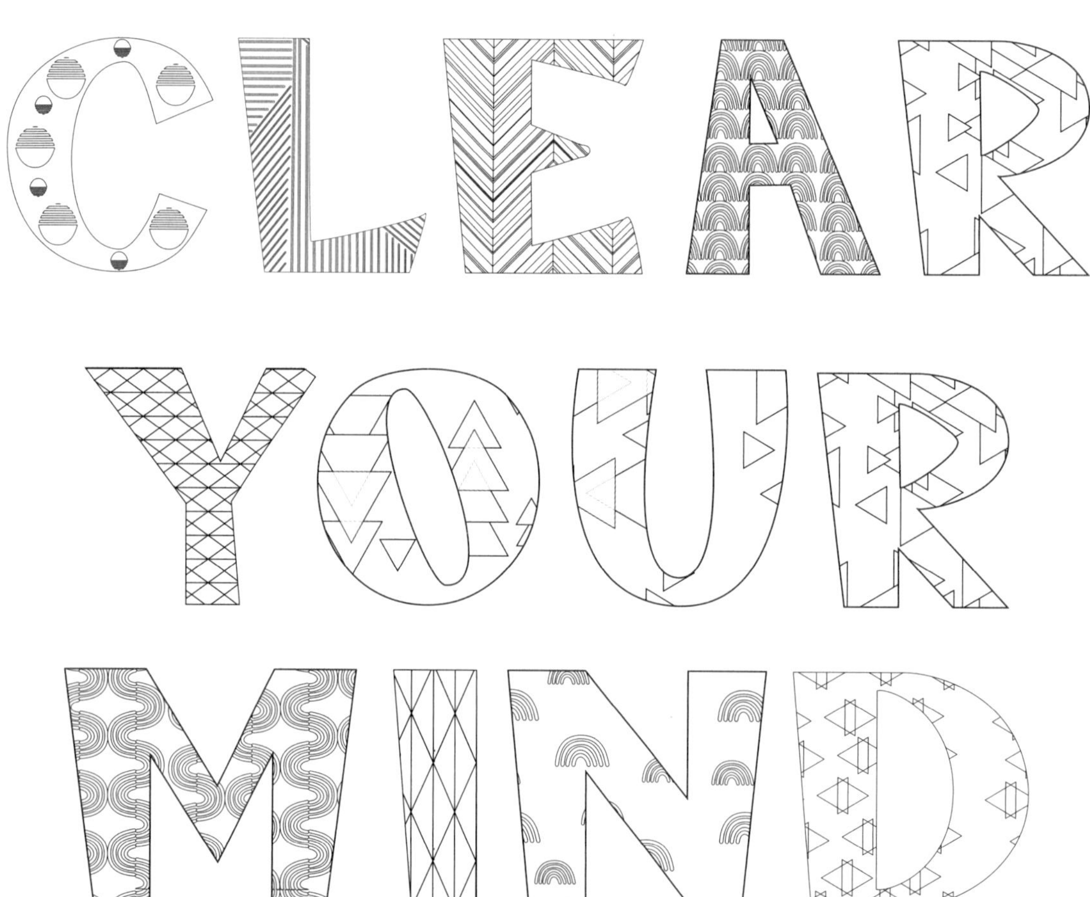
CLEAR
YOUR
MIND

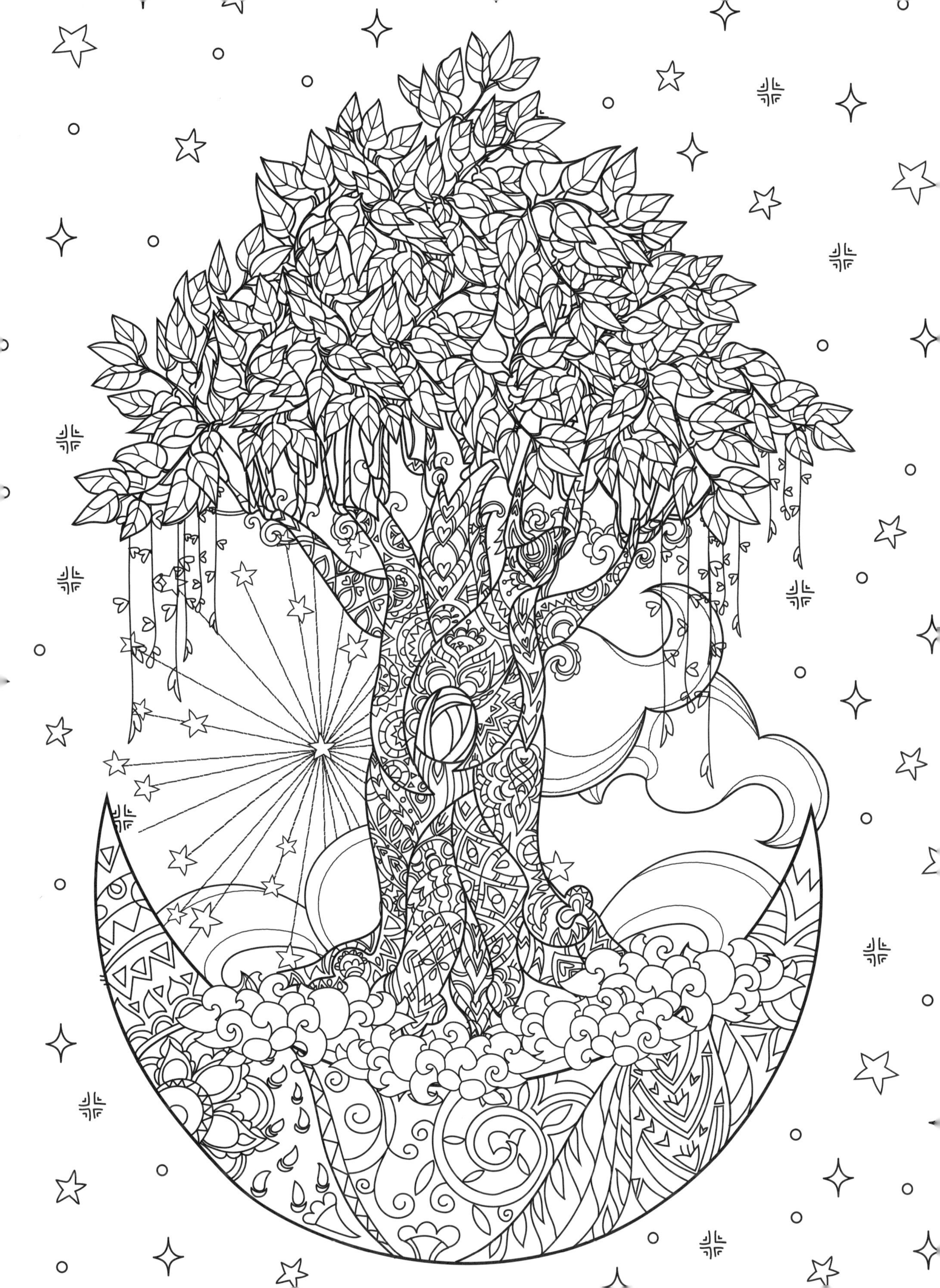

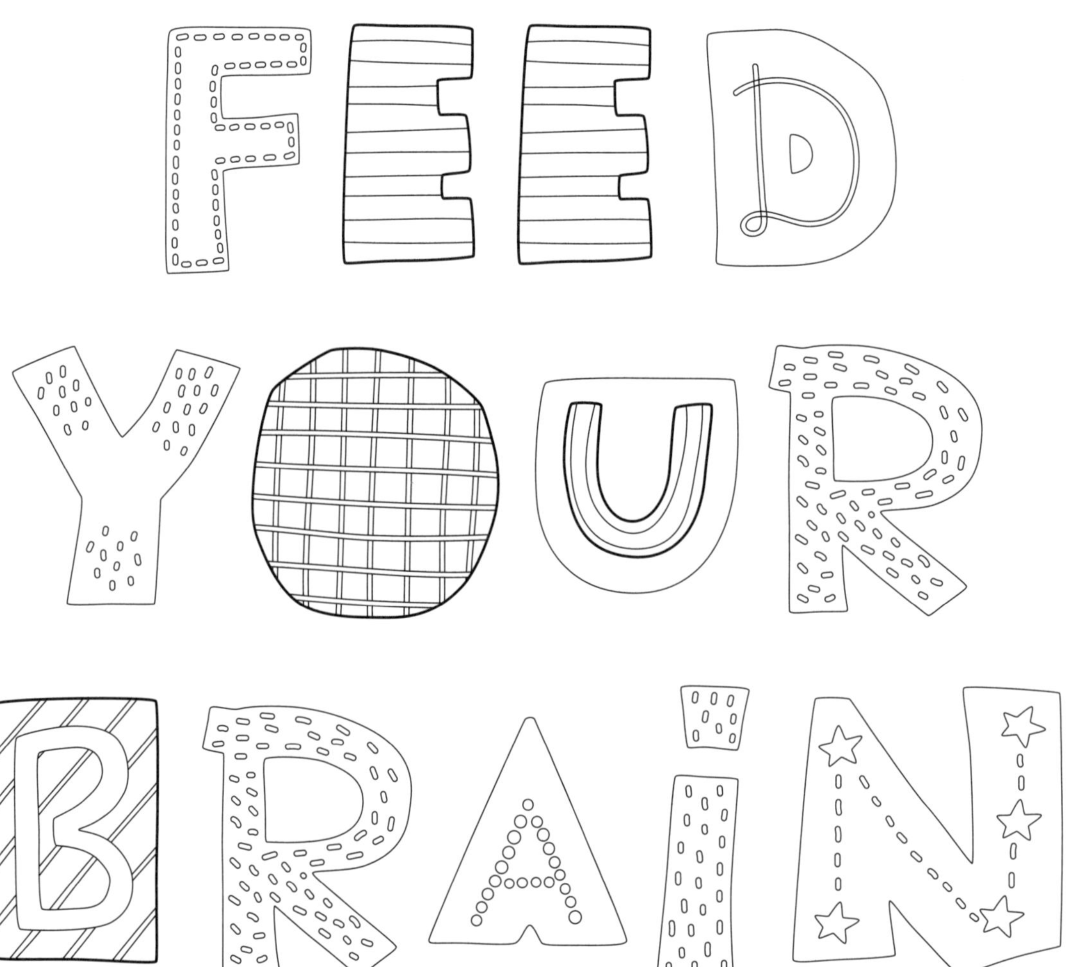
FEED
YOUR
BRAIN

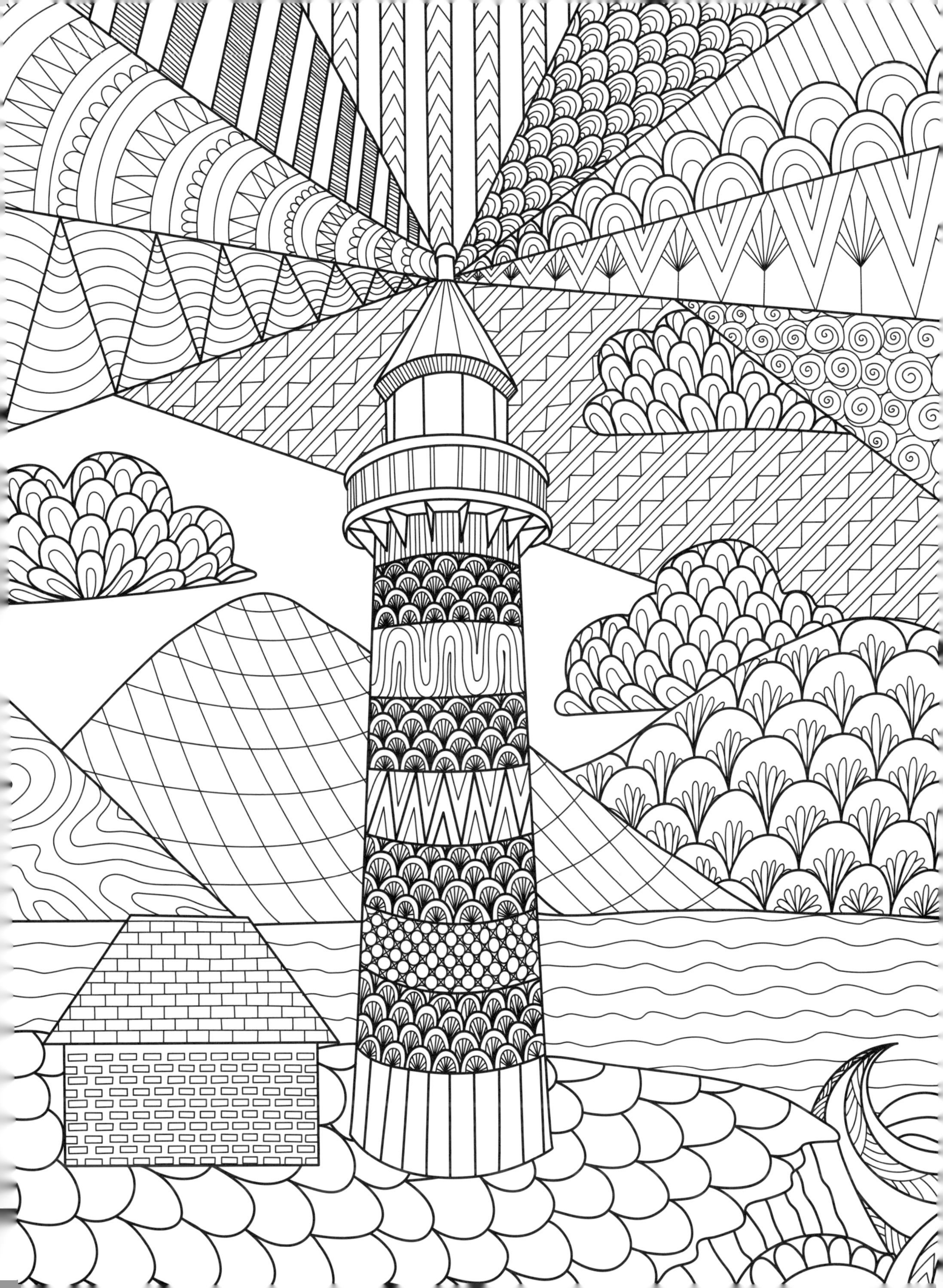

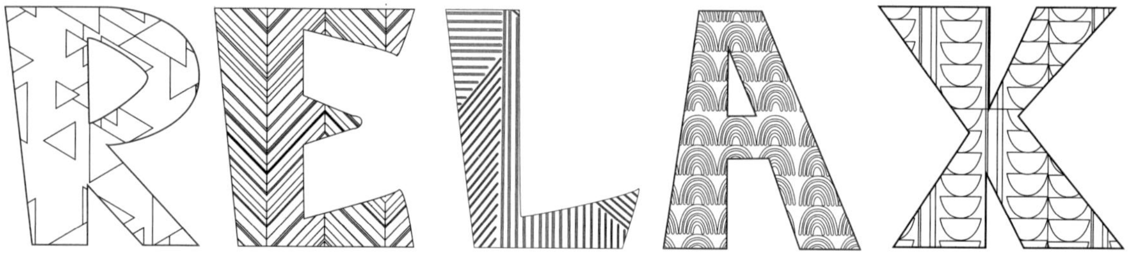
RELAX

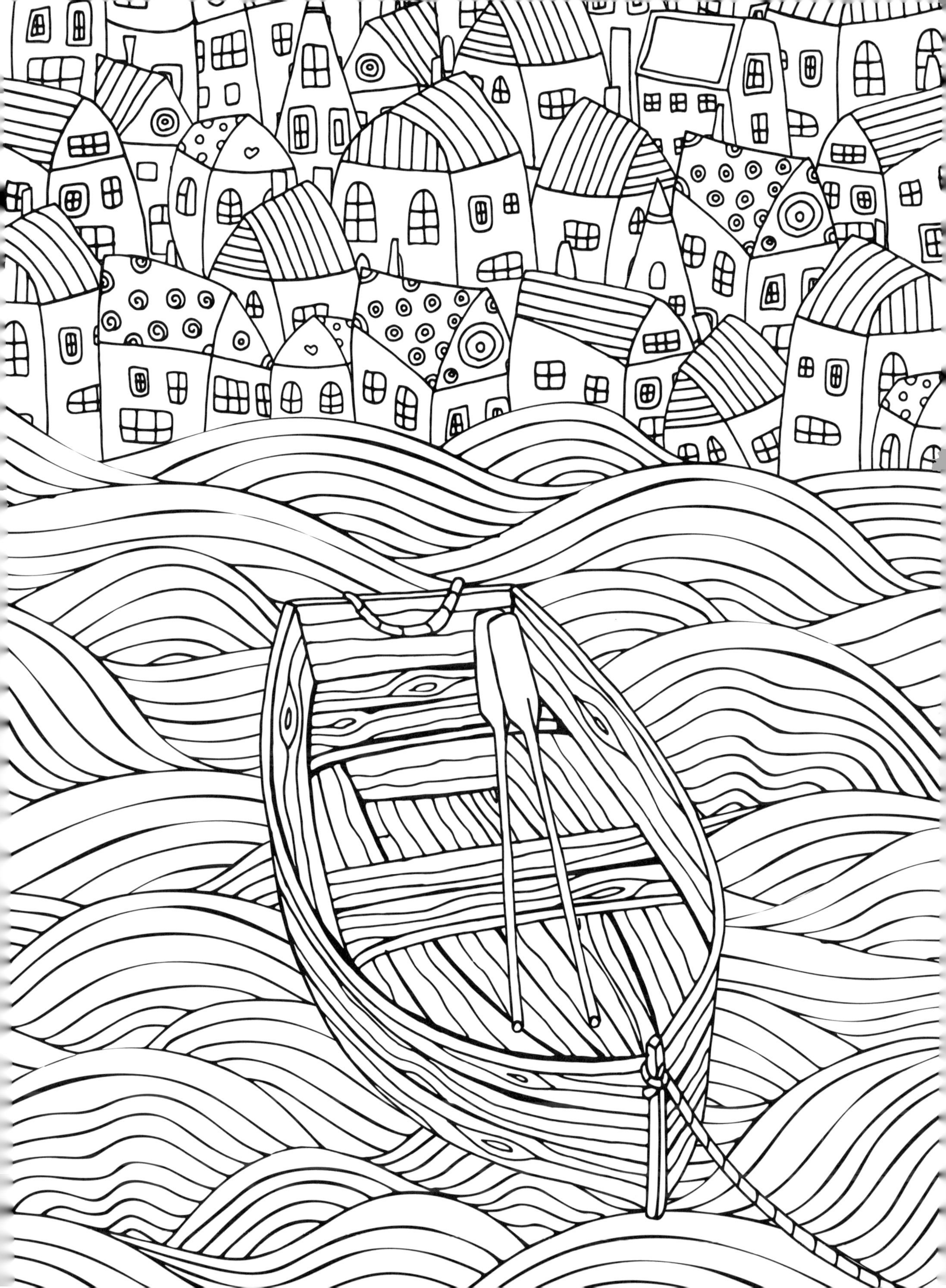

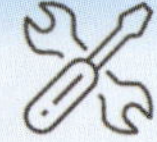

ANXIETY TOOLKIT

Reflect on your journey and make a plan to keep your anxiety at bay.

What could be better? Anxiety is a complex condition. Many people carry it with them for a lifetime; for others, it comes and goes. Hopefully you will feel like you've developed and grown over the course of this book and have become more confident at managing your anxiety. It's an ongoing journey and there will likely still be areas you know you can improve. Use this space to make a note of things you need to continue to work on.

Gather together all your learnings and compile everything you've found helpful in one space. This can be a quick reference guide for you in the future. You should think about the strategies and coping mechanisms, lifestyle modifications, support systems, and treatments that have been most effective.

My best coping strategies

Lifestyle habits that help me

Best people to ask for support

Websites / groups / resources I find useful

Effective treatments or medications

Anything else

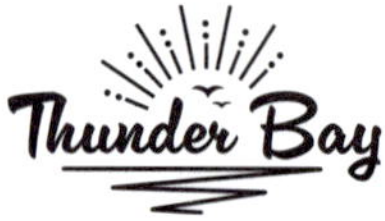

Thunder Bay Press
An imprint of Printers Row Publishing Group
9717 Pacific Heights Blvd, San Diego, CA 92121
www.thunderbaybooks.com • mail@thunderbaybooks.com

Printers Row Publishing Group is a division of Readerlink Distribution Services, LLC.

Thunder Bay Press is a registered trademark of Readerlink Distribution Services, LLC.

Correspondence regarding the content of this book should be sent to Thunder Bay Press, Editorial Department, at the above address.

Thunder Bay Press

Publisher: Peter Norton

Associate Publisher: Ana Parker

Art Director: Charles McStravick

Editor: Dan Mansfield

Future PLC

Editor: Zara Gaspar

Senior Art Editor: Andy Downes

Writers: Edoardo Albert, Cris Andrews, Sarah Bankes, Sophie Barton, Julie Bassett, Rebecca Bradbury, Jo Cole, Natalie Denton, Bee Ginger, Ben Grafton, Rebecca Greig, Alex Hennessy, Faye M Smith

ISBN: 978-1-6672-1266-1

Printed in Heshan, China

First printing, January 2026. LP/01/26

30 29 28 27 26 1 2 3 4 5

Image Credits

All imagery supplied by Getty Images, Adobe Stock, Firefly AI.